Jacinta Nandi

WTF BERLIN

WTF BERLIN

EXPATSPLAINING THE GERMAN CAPITAL

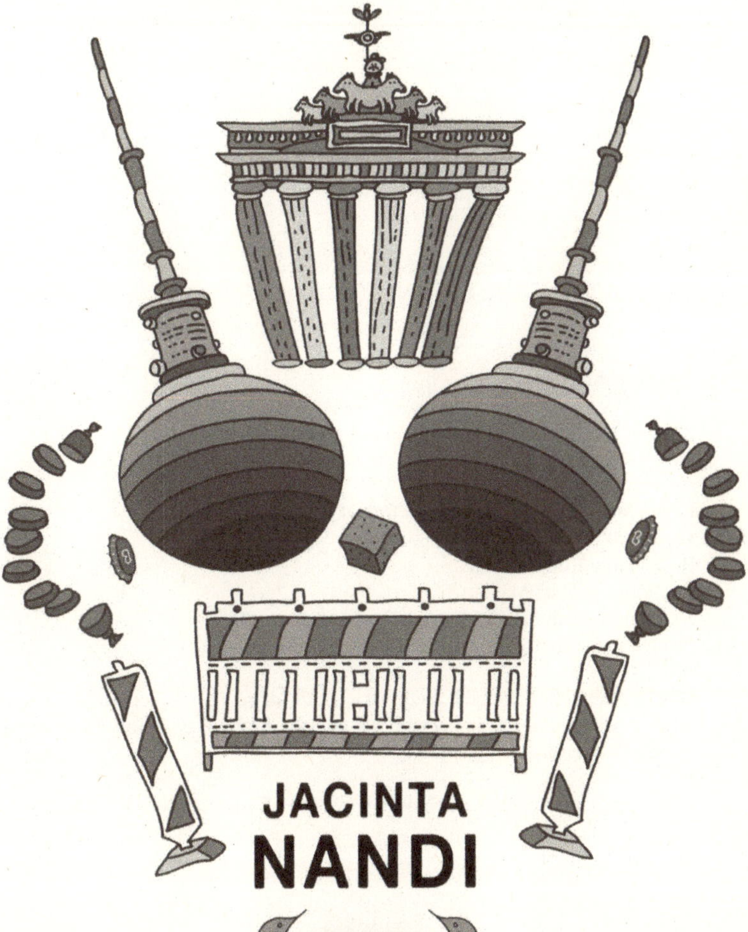

JACINTA
NANDI

SATYR

Dieses Buch wurde klimaneutral auf FSC-zertifiziertem Papier aus nachhaltigen Quellen gedruckt. Die Kaschierfolie des Umschlags ist kompostierbar.

1. Auflage Mai 2022

www.satyr-verlag.de

Cover: Jussi Jääskeläinen | www.kobaia-design.com
Lektorat: Phil Butland, Volker Surmann
Korrektorat: Ruby Russell
Autorenfoto: FluxFM
Druck und Bindung: CPI Books, Clausen & Bosse, Leck
Printed in Germany

Die Deutsche Nationalbibliothek verzeichnet diese Publikation in der Deutschen Nationalbibliografie; detaillierte bibliografische Daten sind im Internet abrufbar über: http://dnb.d-nb.de

ISBN: 978-3-947106-82-0

Content

Introduction: Learn German or Die Trying 9

Chapter One: A is for ...

Abendbrot 13

Abtreibung 16

Annie-Way 18

Anmeldung 20

Chapter Two: B is for ...

Bäckerei versus Backshop 24

Begrüßen 27

Birne 30

Chapter Three: C is for ...

Cringe 33

Corona 35

Chapter Four: D is for ...

Der, die das 40

Daten 42

Denglisch 45

Dosen 47

Chapter Five: E is for

Erziehung 51
Einladen 55

Chapter Six: F is for ...

Fernsehenturm 59
Ficktermin 61

Chapter Seven: G is for ...

Gendern 63

Chapter Eight: H is for ...

Handy 66
Hartz IV 67
Hund 69

Chapter Nine: I is for ...

Impfen 73
Indianer 77
Integration 81

Chapter Ten: J is for ...

Jugendamt 83

Chapter Eleven: K is for ...

Kaltmiete 88
Kartoffel 91
Kirchensteuer 93
Kita 97
Koch 99
Kopftuch 103
Kur 107

Chapter Twelve: L is for ...

Latzhose ... 109

Chapter Thirteen: M is for ...

Migrationshintergrundler ... 111
Mülltrennung ... 117

Chapter Fourteen: N is for ...

Nikolaus ... 121
Nummer ... 123

Chapter Fifteen: O is for ...

Opfer ... 125

Chapter Sixteen: P is for ...

Patriotismus ... 128
Partys ... 134

Chapter Seventeen: Q is for ...

Queen ... 139
Quer ... 140

Chapter Eighteen: R is for ...

Romantik ... 144

Chapter Nineteen: S is for ...

Schwarztee ... 148
Shoppen versus Einkaufen ... 150
Silvester ... 154
Späti ... 157
Spielplatz ... 158
Steile These ... 163

Bonus Chapter: ß is for ...

S-Zett 164

Chapter Twenty: T is for ...

Theater 167

Toastbrot 169

Chapter Twenty-One: U is for ...

Umlaut 172

Unzuverlässig 173

Chapter Twenty-Two: V is for ...

Verwandte 177

Chapter Twenty-Three: W is for ...

Wachsen 181

Westdeutschland 184

Wiebke 189

Chapter Twenty-Four: X is for ...

XL 194

Chapter Twenty-Five: Y is for ...

You: Du, Ihr or Sie 196

Chapter Twenty-Six: Z is for ...

Zecke 201

Zug 201

Epilogue: Why You Should Learn German and
Some Tips on How to 205

Glossary 213

Introduction: Learn German or Die Trying

My friend Tanja and I are out in Neukölln, eating dinner with an American friend of hers who has a PhD from a renowned American university. We know he has a PhD because he mentions this fact every 7.4 seconds, and we know the uni he went to is well-renowned because he mentions that fact every 23.5 seconds. Approximately. Tanya and I both went to bog-standard comprehensives and then studied German at non-renowned British universities. Modern languages are taught at such a basic level in Britain that I sometimes feel my Bachelor's degree is almost of as much value as a *Seepferdchen* certificate.

"I like your girlfriend, Paul," I tell him. He has a younger Polish girlfriend who is funnier and sexier than him. At the very least he should be aware, right?

"Yeah?" he says.

"Yeah," I say. "She's great, articulate, smart ..."

"She's not that articulate," he says. "Her English isn't that great, to be honest. My cousin was over from the States the other week and he said he couldn't understand everything she was saying." I take a breath. "I wouldn't know," I say icily. "I speak to her in German."

Maybe I am too petty for words, but I sit there fuming. The arrogance of English speakers in general – and Americans in particular! It drives me mad! Shortly afterwards the waitress arrives and Paul, of course, orders in English. Why wouldn't he? We're in Neukölln, after all.

"How long have you lived here, Paul?" I ask him innocently.

"Seven years," he says.

"Maybe in another seven you'll be able to order your drinks in German," I say.

"Oh, I could order in German if I wanted to," he answers. "It's just easier to be understood in English."

Look, I get it. You couldn't have much more German-speaking privilege than me: eleven years old when I started learning the language *(Und wie geht's Ihnen, Frau Singh?)*, twelve when I visited Limburg for the first time (I saw *Pretty Woman* dubbed into German and understood everything because I knew it off by heart), and twenty when I moved here.

"Are you going to pack your Oxford Duden dictionary?" my mum asked worriedly.

"Mum, I'm practically fluent!" I yelled confidently. Then I arrived here and tried to order a Currywurst – "Ich spreche kein Englisch!" the guy screamed in my face. I was crestfallen – that wasn't English but practically fluent German, right? What was wrong with him? At Warschauer Straße I bought a *Motz* off a homeless guy and he wished me a nice day like an American. "Even the homeless speak English," I whispered to myself forlornly as I suddenly realised that I wasn't brilliant at German. I wasn't even that good at it – I could just speak a tiny, basic bit of it. *(Entschuldigung, Frau Singh!)* So, I'm not about to judge anyone for not being able to speak this horrifically difficult language. And I know how judgy Germans can be: after twenty years here I basically *am* fluent – but because of my non-white appearance and terrible accent, there's a certain type of German (racist) who doesn't even notice.

But not being able to speak German isn't, in my eyes, something to be smug about. It makes life harder – sometimes it can even be dangerous. I remember after giving birth in 2004 in Urban Krankenhaus. It was the first time I had to pee after having my catheter out, and it felt like I was being sliced open by a blade.

"Mein Pinkel, mein Pinkel!" I called.

"What's wrong, what's wrong?" gasped the nurses.

"Mein Pinkel ist ein Messer!" I announced as they burst out laughing.

"Wir wissen genau, was Sie meinen," they said, and reassured me it was normal.

But the last time I went to my family doctor in Neukölln, the doctor got me to speak to the receptionist, showing me off like I was a dog who'd learnt to curtsey or do a *Hitlergruß*.

"Listen to this," the doctor said. "It's amazing. She can say anything she wants to. She's talking in full sentences," he went on.

"I've been here twenty years," I protested weakly.

I think it's okay to live here for twenty years and still not know your adjectival endings – in fact I think it's a bit *unsolidarisch* with people who work in Dönerläden to get too good at German grammar. And I think it's absolutely okay to watch all your Netflix shows in English. I also think it's okay to become demotivated and lazy when speaking to those German friends whose English is practically perfect and who, let's face it, just want to use you as a free English teacher (hello, Cornelius!).

But it's not okay to judge non-native speakers whose English isn't perfect when you've been living in the country for seven years and still can't order yourself a fucking *Orangensaft*. Come on, man. And now that everyone's streaming all their favourite shows in English, you're not going to teach yourself German through daytime TV or by watching the same episode of *Friends* dubbed into German one million times. The only thing you can do is get yourself back to school – and I don't mean an Ivy League one. The Volkshochschule will do.

Chapter One: A is for …

Abendbrot: Abend *means evening and* Brot *means bread, but if you put them together and look up the word* Abendbrot *in the dictionary, you might get a bit confused. They'll try to tell you it's dinner – or supper. But in British English, at least, it's more like tea –* AbendESSEN *is dinner whereas* AbendBROT *is a light evening meal, normally cold, made up of bread and cheese and salami.*

And when I say light, I really mean LIGHT. There are anorexic fruit flies heavier than German Abendbrot. *It is, quite literally, the Perfect German Housewife's best kept secret.*

Abendbrot: The German Housewife's Best-Kept Secret

I am a bad housewife in more ways than I can count: I hate hoovering, I can't mop, I don't even know how to iron. When I iron something it looks more creased afterwards and has these funny black marks which I don't think are supposed to be there. I once stacked the dishwasher so badly that my ex-boyfriend cried actual tears of actual frustration and true grief. And I think if Marie Kondo watched me folding laundry it would possibly break her.

But when it comes to German *Abendbrot*, I am the Perfect German Housewife. I have that shit *down*.

So, I'm babysitting my lovely friend Florence's kid when my equally lovely little friend Lola comes over. Lockdown has been lifted, but I still want her to sit on the balcony. I know she's been partying loads. Lola is so tiny and perfect – I swear, she is the only person on the planet who actually lost weight over lockdown – and now she looks so perfect and petite and tiny, like a tiny miniature porcelain chimney sweep.

"They change the rules every day," she says mournfully, placing two bottles of Sekt on the table. "It's cold on your balcony, let's just open the balcony doors, then your kitchen is kind of part of the balcony. Oh, I am so confused about the Corona stuff. Are you confused? It's so confusing!"

"It is confusing, isn't it," I say.

"It's exhausting and confusing!" she says. "I don't even know what is allowed or not anymore! Are we allowed to shake strangers' hands? Have sex with our old pre-Corona fuck buddies? Smoke crack together if we disinfect the pipe first? What about ketamine? Is ketamine illegal now?"

"I think, even in non-Corona times, ketamine is not strictly speaking legal. But yeah, it's all so confusing! I think they need to make up some simple rules and let us know what they are and then we can stick to them. I'm not even sure if I should have let you come over when I'm babysitting. Listen, I'm gonna make the kids some Abendbrot, you open the Sekt, okay?"

Abendbrot is probably the greatest trick the Perfect German Housewife ever played on German men/ausländische women, I think, as I get the kids' tea ready. That is, I place two slices of grey bread, one slice of cheese and one slice of salami on the plate. Lola looks over my shoulder.

"Has that kid you're babysitting's mum fucked your ex-boyfriend or something?" she asks, looking at the plate of food I have prepared.

"What?" I say.

"You obviously really hate this woman? You're giving her kid the cheapest, stingiest, most miserable excuse for dinner known to man."

I look at Lola in surprise.

"Lola!" I say. "This is *Abendbrot*! This is German *Abendbrot*! This is good, normal, German *Abendbrot*. This is how you German."

"Oh for fuck's sake, you are so mean about the Germans sometimes."

"No, honestly, this is what German kids get for dinner."

"This is what people in the Bastille got for dinner, more like! At the very fucking least put the two slices of bread on top of each other and call it a fucking sandwich."

"Lola, I am a perfect German housewife, and I would never do anything as outrageously and horrifically un-German as give my kids a sandwich for dinner. Well ... not when we have guests over."

Yep, *Abendbrot* is probably the greatest trick the Perfect German Housewife ever played on German men/ausländische women. If you grab a slice of bread, but actually go to the trouble of chopping up an onion, frying some bacon, getting some turkey ham involved. Or even smearing said bread with something vaguely healthy and interesting like hummus or peanut butter. YOU SLUT YOU LAZY SLUT YOU DISGUSTING WHORE YOU FUCKING ... *AUSLÄNDERIN*.

The brilliance of *Abendbrot* is, the less effort you put in, the more German and perfect it becomes.

Now, for example, in my home country, England, a country famously famous for being bad at cooking, we think the mums who make easy dinners – bangers and mash, say, or beans on toast – we think THEY are the lazy housewives! Whereas the women who actually make complicated, tasty, delicious meals like lasagne or quiche are the good mothers – and proper housewives.

But Germany is like opposite world and everyone (except Lola) knows that the Perfect German Housewife makes a perfect Abendbrot: two slices of bread, two slices of tired, slightly wilted cucumber (you should try to buy your cucumbers at the supermarket already on the verge of exhaustion to get the real Abendbrot feeling), one slice of cheese, one slice of salami.

One thing I'd like to see: a Nigella Lawson German Abendbrot reaction video. Or how about if we forced Nigella Lawson to make a German Abendbrot herself? I think this would be literally torture for her. I reckon at the last moment she'd go crazy and start smearing the bread with organic goose fat, smashing up avocados and throwing smarties at all the kids.

***

Abtreibung: *So,* Treiben *is a super weird German word. It means something like drive, but not in a car, right. The drive in what's driving you. But sometimes it just means do. The complicated thing is when you* übertreiben, *you're overdoing things, but you might be exaggerating – when you* untertreiben, *you're kind of playing things down – and when you* abtreiben, *you're having an abortion. It sounds really dark and cruel, like you can imagine DDR doctors using old-fashioned knives and stuff.*

A kind of euphemism for abortion is Abbruch. *The way I always think of it is: abortion is* Abtreibung *and* Abbruch *is termination.*

Abortions are hugely taboo in Germany, even in Berlin – slightly less taboo in East Germany and East Berlin than in the West, but still super taboo. The thing is, Germans, like the perverted weirdo weird perverts that they are, don't actually look down on women who have abortions because they think they are sluts or that sex is dirty and disgusting and shameful and stuff. Germans actually just seem to think sex is this thing you do sometimes, kind of by accident. But the thought of a woman being enough of a disorganised hot mess to forget to take a pill at the exact same time each day horrifies them.

Don't forget that abortions are actually officially illegal in Germany, and it's only just been made legal to "advertise" – i.e. inform people – of the fact that you carry out abortions if you are a gynaecologist.

Now, while it's true that they don't actually prosecute women who have an abortion before the twelfth week (which I find a super early date to decide by, by the way) it being officially a crime means that it is really hard to get one, or talk about it openly.

We spend a lot of time in Germany worrying about how fucked-up other countries are, and sometimes it means we don't notice the ways in which Germany is a fucked-up place to live. The abortion stuff is super fucked-up over here. White German men assume it's easy to get one, but they don't want to hear any details.

Abortion, Abortion!

I'm super pregnant and at a new gynaecologist on the Schönhauser Allee. People make jokes about how you can't be a "little bit" pregnant, but it's not true, huh? Loads of people who get a faint line on their pregnancy test end up miscarrying. And I, right now, here, right now, I AM A LOT PREGNANT.

I look like a whale. I feel like a hippo. People treat me like a walrus. I waddle around like a penguin.

My ankles are swollen up like soft, fleshy balloons. I feel like my bones have melted inside me.

In the form the lady has given me I have to tick which pregnancy this is. This is my third pregnancy. I had two abortions before I came to Germany. I feel like lying on the form, but I worry the doctor will be able to somehow "tell" – possibly by looking at my AOK medical records, and, slightly less possibly, but even more horrifically, by looking at my vagina? So I tick third on the box, hand my forms in and go back to my seat in the waiting room. The waiting room is full of pregnant women, expectant mothers. There's pink carpet, beige walls, and sepia pictures of mums breastfeeding their babies everywhere. It's expectant mummy hour at the gyno.

The doctor's receptionist comes into the waiting room and says to me, loudly and clearly: "These two pregnancies here, how did they end?"

"Pardon?" I say.

"Did your two previous pregnancies end in miscarriage, abortion or birth?" she asks.

"Abortion," I whisper through the side of my mouth.

She shouts loudly: "TWO ABORTIONS!" *Zwei Abbrüche*!

I nod.

The receptionist leaves the waiting room, and it's just me, fat like a whale, a load of pregnant German women, and the sepia pictures. I start studying *Bild der Frau* like I'm really into it. Maybe I should change my name to Jacinta Two Abortions Nandi, I think. It has a nice ring to it.

* * *

Annie-Way: Annie-Way *is the way Germans in the early 2000s (the* Nullerjahre, *as they would put it) pronounced anyway. As with almost all the best* Denglisch *terms, the way they used it was slightly, ever-so-slightly, wrong.*

Denglish is Like Bindweed

Denglisch – I personally think the most annoying thing about Denglisch is not the way it crowds out and destroys Proper German like some kind of disgustingly destructively violently vandalistic *Unkraut* (Denglisch is like the grey, violent, American-style "squirrels" which invaded Britain after World War II and Proper German is like the sweet, innocent, totally cute, actually-look-like-squirrels-and not-bastard-rats-with-fluffy-tails-type squirrels which died out in Britain, but still, gorgeously, live here. Every time I see a cute orange squirrel I say to my son, darkly, all the squirrels I grew up with were ugly, I only saw this kind in books, look how cute it is.) Denglisch starves Proper German out. I once sat in *Tropical Islands* for two hours, trying desperately to remember what the Proper German for lifeguard was. In the end, I went to my locker, took out my phone, and googled it. (It's *Bademeister*, or *Rettungsschwimmer*, by the way.) I once asked everyone in a hotel in Mecklenburg-Vorpommern what they said for *einchecken* and *auschecken* in the DDR. Honestly, the Denglisch terms take up the space in your brain where the Proper German should go, that was some serious Mandela Effect shit, yeah, like as if the aliens had been wiping everyone's memories most effectively. A lot of people said, 100 per cent certain, "It was always *ein-* and *auschecken*!" But some people whispered vaguely: "I ... don't ... know. It couldn't have been *auschecken* ... could it? Could it? What did we used to say? We must have said something ... I think I knew it once."

DENGLISCH literally KILLING the Proper German in your head is very, very, very annoying – but it's not the most annoying thing.

The most annoying thing about Denglisch is, without a doubt, when Germans throw a Denglisch word into a German sentence for no reason whatsoever – and you have no idea if they are doing it especially for you because they know you are a native speaker, or if this is A New Thing People Say.

There's a poetry slammer organiser who always says to me: "Du bist so *charming* auf der Bühne!" – have checked with others, this is just for me. It's not A Thing. But how the fuck are you meant to know? "Das ist ja irgendwie doch super *niiiiiiice*!" THIS IS A THING. "I know, I know," inexplicably plonked into the sentence: THIS IS ALSO A THING.

And *Annie-Way*? This isn't, and don't ask me why, a thing anymore. But it was for ages – right up until, like 2009, I'd say – and it was really fucking annoying. In the middle of a sentence, for no reason whatsofuckingever, out of nowhere, "*Annie-way*!"

* * *

Anmeldung: Anmeldung *means registration, and* Abmeldung *means deregistration. But Germans register for things more than English speakers do – you have to register with the library, register at the gym, register at the nursery. And they definitely deregister more. I feel like in other countries you can just stop doing something, and then it's over, but in Germany you always have to* abmelden. *But one of the weirdest things about Germany is undoubtedly that everyone in the entire country has to* anmelden *with the government – and nobody seems to mind!*

Achtung, Achtung, Anmeldung, Anmeldung!

Germans love privacy and stuff, but weirdly don't mind the government having a huge database of where everyone in the country lives.

"Are you still sleeping with that old boy? The one who didn't know that Wales wasn't part of England?" I ask my tiny friend Lola, who can sometimes have really bad taste in men, especially old men.

"Of course not!" she says, outraged. "I've been socially distancing! I'm only having casual sex with people I actually like!"

I nod.

It's the first time I've seen her since the half-hearted German lockdown ended. We're sitting by the Paul-Linke-Ufer and not sharing two separate bottles of cider. I keep thinking I see Prof. Dr. Christian Drosten walk past, so I smile. But it's just a vaguely sexy, fairly sad German guy walking with a bike. I have to admit, it's great to be out. I always thought I was a hermit, but after six weeks stuck inside, I actually truly enjoy going out again.

It's a great feeling.

The constant, slight boredom – a constant, slight panic I wasn't having fun and would rather be at home on Facebook – has disappeared. I now know I *do* want to go out sometimes.

"He really is old," she says. "He's an old man. He smells old. He feels old. He feels wrinkly. His waist seems like it has arthritis."

"I was surprised by how old he was," I say, diplomatically.

"You know how you notice how old he is?" she says. "He still says *polizeiliche Anmeldung*. Have you ever noticed that? Old people are always saying *polizeiliche Anmeldung*?"

"What?" I say.

"You never noticed? Old people think it's called *polizeiliche Anmeldung*. I guess in the olden days – like in the sixties and stuff – you had to go and *anmelden* at the police station? You never noticed?"

I stare at Lola, horrified. I had, in fact, not noticed that. I had *very much not* noticed that. And I'll tell you something else I hadn't noticed. I had not noticed that young people don't call it a *polizeiliche Anmeldung* anymore.

And I will tell you another thing I hadn't noticed: that I am an old person now, my skin wrinkled, my vagina crumpled and crinkly like the pages of an old, dusty bible. My body is so old and ancient that when Germany's top euthanasia-ist talks about letting old fogies die of Corona to reduce overpopulation, it is, basically, me she is talking about. I am old now and death is, quite literally, just around the corner.

I have been anmelding in Germany for twenty years. When I arrived, I was petrified of the idea. I thought it was, basically, Stasi as fuck. The police had a big database with the name and address of everyone in the fucking country? What? I channelled Kafka, registered myself and felt scared and petrified and horrified the whole time I was doing it.

I've got used to it now, though. This is what twenty years in Germany has done to me. I now often forget that you don't need to register with the authorities in Britain. To be honest, a part of me, a tiny part of me, still thinks it's weird and oppressive. Why are we slagging China or North Korea off? But 95 per cent of me thinks it's pretty practical and useful. During that awful year after the Brexit referendum, when Polish teenagers were being asked to submit twenty years of electricity bills with their names on them or leave the country immediately, it seemed to me that the only possible solution would be to implement some kind of *Anmeldung* system. If you are going to be Stasi as fuck, at least do it right.

But what about all the white Germans who think the Corona app is creepy? Or that *Impfpflicht* is somehow a terrible human rights abuse? Or those weirdos who think it's child abuse to put picture of your kid blowing out their birthday cake candles on Instagram? I don't get it. If I was 100 per cent on board with *Anmeldung* – with being literally legally required to tell the *fucking government* where I lived – I wouldn't care about my privacy in any other way. But I guess, despite twenty years here, I'll never really be German.

Chapter Two: B is for ...

Bäckerei versus Backshop: Bäckerei *is the German word for bakery, and it says something about British bakers that the first time I went to a* Bäckerei *in Germany, the German guy I was with told me that they didn't even bake the bread on the premises – and I thought for the first time in my life "Oh yeah, the word bakery must come from baking!"*

Backshops *are cheapo Berlin-style bakers. I love them. German people in Berlin are always complaining that real bakeries are dying out and you can't get good bread anywhere and stuff like that. And I feel for them, I really do – but not enough to go to a real bakery.*

Baking My Way Through Lockdown One

This is the kind of mother I would have liked to have been during the lockdown: calm, conscientious, relaxed, loving – and good at baking. Yes, good at baking – but not in a smug, smarmy sort of way, oh no. I wish I was good at baking in a sloppy, vegan, witchy, almost-but-not-quite lesbian kind of way. This is the kind of person, the kind of mother, I would like to have been.

The kind of mums who are good at baking in a smug way are sensible, practical people – good at baking, good at homeschooling, too. They baked scones, muffins, brownies, things like that. The kind of witchy women I admire fucked the homeschooling in the mouth with a broomstick and made weird, vegan stuff – Indian scones or zucchini muffins or gluten-free, 100 per cent kakao brownies. I despise people who bake in a middle-class, show-offy kind of a way, and want to be like people who bake weird vegan stuff. Oh, and sourdough bread! I think I admire people who bake sourdough bread. I don't know what it is and can't be bothered to google, but I think if I knew what it was, I would want to bake some. A lot.

But this is the kind of mother I am, and this is how I bake during the Half-hearted German Lockdown: I scroll recipes on my phone for inspiration, recipes for scones, muffins and brownies. I look at the list of ingredients, and then half-heartedly scour my Corona-Hamster-Schrank for flour and baking powder. I don't bother weighing anything, and decide to use *Traubenzucker* instead of *Feinzucker,* and tell myself that if the thing we're baking comes out more like chocolate scones, we'll call them chocolate scones – that's a thing, right? – and if they come out more like muffins, we'll call them muffins, and nobody will be any the wiser.

"Maybe," I say to Baby Leo, my assistant baker, "we will have invented a new type of chocolate goodie, the scuffin."

"Wow!" he says wisely, and then runs to the kitchen wall and presses a chocolate hand against the whiteness, and makes a perfect handprint. My heart sinks when I see this and I look at the goo we have created, and remember baking powder.

"I forgot to put baking powder in!" I say to Baby Leo.

"Wow!" he says.

"No, it's bad," I say. "It's bad Mummy forgot."

"Oh no!" he whispers. "Oh dear!" I think he might be a TV presenter when he grows up, there's this gorgeous simplicity to his emotions which reminds me, kind of, of Holly Willoughby or the lady who's always on with Piers Morgan.

We put the chocolate blobs on a tin and push it in the oven.

"Wow!" Baby Leo says magnificently. I wash his hands clean and try to remove the choccie hand stain from the perfect white wall. I take him out onto the balcony.

Baby Leo starts playing dinosaurs and I scroll Facebook, feeling guilty for even having a balcony in the first place.

I watch a boy I know gingerly removing the crime scene tape the landlords put over the slide in our courtyard playground and have a sneaky, slide down. I don't blame the kids for sneaking onto the playground equipment, I don't blame parents for struggling. But it makes me mad that we could all bear to not go to playground when it was cold – but we can't avoid the playground for a few months to save people's lives?

The timer on my phone goes off.

"I think our muffins are ready," I say to Baby Leo. "Or scones. We'll see what they most look like. Maybe scuffins. Maybe we'll have invented a new type of food. Maybe I'll get rich. And we can move to Potsdam!"

I pull the tray out of the oven and the scuffins I have baked are pretty much inedible. Maybe I should tell everyone they're rock cakes, I say to myself. No, even if chocolate rock cakes were a thing, these are disgusting.

Baby Leo bites into one and announces, cheerfully: "AUWA!"

"They're not very yummy, are they?" I say.

"Cookies. Is. Nicht. Yummy. Cookies. Is. Auwa. Meine. Mouth."

"I know exactly what you mean," I say. I'll wait for them to cool down and throw them on the compost heap, I think. And then we'll put a bit of telly on. This lockdown. It won't last forever.

* * *

Begrüßen: Begrüßen *means greeting each other, and it's a much more serious affair over here than in the UK, at least. You also have to, if you're on the phone to someone you know, send them* ganz doll schöne Grüße. *This is much nicer than just telling them you said hi, but isn't QUITE as nice as giving them your love. I feel like maybe in the olden days British people greeted each other like Germans do – but nowadays it's all giving love or saying hello – or maybe even saying nothing at all!*

Important German Greetings Etiquette: Greet Each Other in the Coldest Voice Imaginable, and Then Say Absolutely Nothing to Each Other Ever Again as Long as You Both Shall Live

Have you guys noticed how, whenever you enter a German doctor's waiting room, you have to say "Guten Tag!" to everyone in the unfriendliest, coldest voice ever, do a small clicky nod of your chin, keep your mouth shut tight like they are your mortal enemies, avoid eye contact, and then sit down in ABSOLUTE SILENCE?

This is known in Germany as *Grüßen* – greeting people – and apparently it's a very, very, very, very important tradition. "Guten Tag!" Bark it out like as if you're a *Kontrolleur* on the U8 on a Saturday night. Avoid eye contact. You don't want any actual contact with these people. Make sure, whatever you do, you don't smile. DO NOT SMILE. Please, please, please for the love of God, don't smile. And then sit down in ABSOLUTE silence. *Grüßen* has nothing to do with actually wanting to speak to people or smile at them or spark up conversation or be friendly with them in any way. It's just this inexplicable thing you do, which inexplicably, is incredibly important.

When my first son was little, another mum at the nursery came up to me and said: “Can I ask you a question?” I don’t want to poke fun at her for doing this, it was obvious to me that something was really bothering her, that this conversation was really important to her, that this was something that had laid heavy on her heart.

“Yeah!” I said.

“Why don’t you greet me?” she asked, flushing. “Have I offended you in some way?”

I stared at her. It was the first time in my life that I realised, that in some ways, English speakers can seem rude to Germans. It was a kind of epiphany moment, I guess. I almost felt guilty, and I definitely felt kind of touched that she had confronted me for this perceived slight.

“Erm?” I said, as politely as possible. “Because I don’t know you?”

She gulped at that, and I really did feel guilty for a moment.

“I think if our kids attend the same nursery, the least we can do is say hello to each other in the cloakroom!”

“Okay,” I said. And from that day on, I’ve been grüßing like a fucking pro.

I only got in trouble one other time for it, years and years later, at a kind of like BnB/cheapo hotel in Mecklenburg-Vorpommern (Pomerania? Lol). A kind of scary-looking white guy, not scary-looking enough to be an actual Nazi, but still a tough guy, barked at me at breakfast:

“In Germany we greet each other at breakfast!”

“Not in hotels?” I exclaimed back. *“Das wäre* echt *übertrieben!”*

I have lived here, as I always annoyingly say, for one million, zillion, SQUILLION years but to be honest I’ve never really understood the whole *Grüßen* thing. Why do we greet each other at the doctor's, but not in the tram? Why do we greet each other and then sit there in silence? What's the point? Why do we greet each other but not smile and joke like we're glad to be alive? People in England will not greet each other for hours or days or weeks or months before anyone gets offended – but once you do greet each other you have this weird crazy totally strange thing called AN ACTUAL CONVERSATION afterwards.

It's also kinda weird to realise that Germans find us rude. We're so used to finding them rude – "You look much older recently, Jacinta, when I met you, you looked young for your age, now you look about seven years older than you really are, what do you think it is? Your thyroid problems?" – that we completely forget that they might find us rude. But they do. Talking loudly on the bus, tram or train. This is, I think, as rude in Germany as fucking on the train would be in English-speaking countries. Facebook-video-chatting on the Deutsche Bahn. I once was scrolling on my phone and my auntie Facebook-rang me and I answered and whispered: "I can't talk, I am on the train, you're not supposed to Facebook call on German trains, it's really rude here!" And when I looked up the whole carriage was grinning away, glowing with approval. They were proud of me, they were proud of what they had turned me into. Eating on the train. Eating stinky kebabs on the train. Laughing loudly on the train. Germans like their trains to be silent and odourless. They are, I will admit, a tiny bit hypocritical about this – a group of male football fans gets on, drinking loads of beer, munching down on smelly fast food and chanting football songs, and the train just bristles slightly. If you're not speaking German or, heaven forbid, unterwegs with kids, they'll be delighted to show you their disapproval. But still. There are things we find kind of okay that they find rude, and it's surprising to discover that the rudest people in THE UNIVERSE can find you rude.

The thing I really will never, ever, ever understand about the greeting thing though is this: if someone doesn't greet you, instead of getting offended, why wouldn't you just greet them first instead of confronting them about it? Nobody ever has ever said hello to anyone and not got a hello back, not even Donald Trump and people like that. I don't get it. I literally have never understood this. And to be honest, I kind of suspect I never will.

* * *

Birne: Birne *is a pear, but a* Glühbirne *is a lightbulb. Germans, even really old ones, don't really think avocados are pears, by the way. And: a bulb you do gardening with is just a* Blumenzwiebel *– a flower onion.*

Let There Be Light!

The weirdest thing about Germany, of all the weird things, is that when you rent a place they don't just take the light bulbs out – but all the light fixtures, too. You have to literally pay electricians or bribe *Hausmeisters** you once fucked to connect the wires together and stuff. I have no idea WHY people do this? I wonder if they think it's a fire hazard, but it would be weird for these people who put actual candles on Christmas trees, throw fireworks at grannies' heads from balconies every New Years Eve, and often lock the front door to blocks of flats to suddenly, suddenly suddenly care about fire hazards?

"Jacinta!" My friend Lola is on the phone. You know things

* The correct plural of "Hausmeister" is also "Hausmeister". — German editor

are bad when a tiny millennial pixie rings you up on the actual telephone.

"Has someone died?" I ask frantically.

"No, but the people at my squat made me move rooms," she whispers dramatically. "And now they are bullying me."

"How are they bullying you?"

"THEY TOOK THE LIGHTS OUT OF MY ROOM!" she wails. "Not just the light bulbs – but the actual light bit you attach the bulb too. Like why would you ever do this to anyone? I wouldn't do this to my worst enemy."

"Try not to take things personally," I say. "It's just a thing Germans do. I don't know why they do it. I think they think electric light is an incredibly new invention and maybe the person moving into their old flat might prefer candles or lanterns or something."

"Don't take it personally?" Lola is choking and sobbing desperately on the phone. "I AM SITTING HERE IN THE FUCKING DARK BECAUSE THESE PEOPLE HATE ME MORE THAN I HATE DONALD TRUMP!"

"Look, I mean this in the most feminist way possible," I say. "You need to phone a man who lives near you, not a single mum who lives at least an hour away. Best of all, a man you slept with once. They need to put a red wire on a red wire and a green wire on a green wire or something. It actually seems like it's not an impossible thing to do, but I have no idea why Germans, who pride themselves on being efficient, don't just leave the lights up for the next person moving in, on the off-chance that they, you know, might like to see at night-time and stuff."

"Which man should I phone? Tell me who."

"An electrician or Hausmeister you fucked once will normally do it."

"What about just a nice friendly man who might want to help me out of the goodness of his heart? Like what about Irish Stu?"

"No, not Irish Stu," I say. "He came over to do mine and electrocuted himself. I still feel guilty about it, to be honest."

But not as guilty as I would feel if I had taken the fucking lights out of the flat I was moving out of for no fucking reason whatsoever.

Chapter Three: C is for …

Cringe: *The German word for shame/embarrassment is* schämen *– or* sich schämen. Ich schämte mich *means I was ashamed or I was embarrassed. So "I dropped a bottle of red wine in the supermarket, God, it was so embarrassing!" could be translated as "Ich ließ eine Flasche Rotwein im Supermarkt runterfallen – Gott, wie ich mich geschämt habe!"*

And there's a BRILLIANT German word for when someone else's behaviour is so embarrassing that you feel ashamed FOR them: fremdschämen. *If you ever write a tweet people disagree with a lot, bitchy Germans will quote-tweet it and write:* "Fremdschämen pur". *It's how we feel about Donald Trump, how we feel about Boris Johnson and Nigel Farage:* Fremdschämen pur. *(It is also, if we are honest, often said of women whose only crime is to have had a bit too much plastic surgery and gelled-up nails, but that's misogyny for you.)*

So, I actually thought that fremdschämen *was going to be one of those beautiful German words, beautiful, clever, perfect, achingly perfect German words that enter the English language. You know the kind of words I mean,* Schadenfreude *or* Zeitgeist. *But what has happened instead? Instead the English word "cringe" got voted "Jugendwort des Jahres" at the end of 2021 – and all my dreams evaporated into thin air. CRINGE!*

One of the biggest misconceptions about Denglisch, I feel, is that these Denglisch additions to the language are completely unnecessary. That they rob German of nuance, rather than adding to it. I think people who claim this have a very simplistic understanding of language, or sometimes just aren't that good at speaking German, to be honest. It's just untrue that the Denglisch word happy *– pronounced* häppy *– is interchangeable with* glücklich *or that* Schminke *has been ousted by Make-Up. What Denglisch does is add nuance to German – "Ich war ganz häppy" means something like, approximately "I was fleetingly glad for a moment" or maybe even "I was temporarily relieved that my luck had changed!"*

However, and don't judge me too much for this, no matter how hard I try, I don't really understand the difference between cringe *and* fremdschämen. *German friends have tried to explain it to me. Obviously,* cringe *is more slangy and* fremdschämen *sounds more "seriös". Maybe also the cringe you feel when you cringe is slightly more superficial? But I think the biggest difference is in the way the word actually works – Donald Trump's embarrassing tweets, Annalena Baerbock's painfully bad English, they will make you* fremdschämen *but they actually ARE cringe, in the same way that ham is food, or postcards are souvenirs.*

I'd still like fremdschämen *to be used in English. We so need this word.*

Peinlich

I feel like Germans find embarrassment more embarrassing than we Brits do, although I am not 100 per cent sure about this. Maybe they just find different things embarrassing?

I once dropped a bottle of red wine in Kaufland. It exploded all over the floor, Jackson Pollocking approximately two thirds of the aisle we were in.

"That was *peinlich*," my son said to me. He was about eight, and I thought he just didn't know the word embarrassing yet, and was mixing the languages up, something which, you know, is pretty normal for a bilingual kid to do.

"That was embarrassing," I corrected him.

"No," he corrected me back. "It wasn't embarrassing. It was *peinlich*. Very, very, VERY embarrassing."

"Oh," I said.

"*Peinlich* is very, very, very embarrassing," he explained. "And embarrassing is *ein bisschen peinlich*."

"You think?" I said, mulling it over in my head.

"I know," he said sternly.

Bilingual kids are almost always right about this kind of stuff, I find. Almost always. My son's theory that *Obst* = boring fruit like apples and pears whereas *Früchte* = delicious red fruits like strawberries and cherries turned out to be wrong (*Obst* is always edible, but *Früchte* doesn't have to be). But generally, bilingual kids are almost always right and their Ausländer parents are almost always wrong. It's a bit embarrassing really.

* * *

Corona: *For some reason, Germans prefer saying* Corona *to* Co*vid. In the UK, nobody ever says anyone has Corona – they talk about how terrible Corona is, and how much they hate it – but when anyone catches the dreaded lurgy, they're ill with Covid.*

Germans prefer to say Corona *to Covid when talking about the actual illness, I think. And there's a certain sullen defiance to their tones when some people say it:* "Koronaaaaah ..." *that makes it sound like they don't really think it's a real virus!*

I actually decided it was time for me to make some new German friends – I have no idea why I decided to do this, but I just felt like maybe it was time for some new blood in my friendship circle.

So I went out to a German single mums' breakfast, aka *Alleinerziehende-Wochenend-Frühstück.*

The mum I liked best was an intellectual German mum called Kristin, the mum I liked second best was a kind of hippy German mum called Natascha. The rest of the mums were boring and I don't mean in that nice, friendly, nice, boring, British mum kind of way, I mean, and this is probably the most internalised misogynistic thing I will ever say in my entire life, UNBEARABLY BORING IN THAT REALLY FUCKING UNBEARABLY BORING GERMAN MUM WAY and I didn't want to speak to them at all. It kind of reminded me why I don't actually need any new friends and that I'm happiest of all in front of my laptop, arguing with strangers on Facebook or skyping with my dear old mum. Still, I guess a ratio of two out of fifteen ain't bad.

"I thought I had Corona in the week," I said. "On Wednesday. I had all the symptoms, except for a higher temperature. I had diarrhoea. Then I puked. Then I had a dry cough. Then I was shaking and shivering. I felt lethargic. My muscles ached. I had all the symptoms. I feel better now, though, so I must've been wrong."

"I'm not worried about Corona at all," said Kristin, the German intellectual.

"I wasn't worried!" I said. This is, by the way, a blatant lie – a *Lüge, glatter* than Keira Knightley's botoxed forehead. I was desperately trying to ring the hotline, which wasn't even fucking ringing, and weeping to myself, panicked, worried, desperate, despairing, because I was certain I had Corona and would need to be quarantined and I would miss my 40th birthday, and me and my boys were all alone in Germany and nobody cared and what if the virus had mutated and now was deadly for 39-year-olds, that would be just my luck wouldn't it? In between crying and panicking I went and puked a few times, and everyone I knew on Facebook told me to chillax because it was only killing old people and people with cancer and I wasn't even 40 yet and so probably wouldn't die anyway.

"I just wanted to know if I should be tested or not. But I couldn't get through to anyone on the hotline. Then I talked to the Krankenkasse people, and they said they wouldn't test me anyway, I've had no contact with anyone who's had it and my temperature wasn't high enough."

"It's not a serious problem," the intellectual mum said.

"It's not a serious problem?" I asked.

"No, you only die of it if you're old or have cancer," she said. "That's what all these people who are panicking don't understand."

"Erm, yeah," I said. Nothing makes me feel less like a German intellectual than the German intellectuals' extreme indifference to Corona. It makes me feel like a British DUMBO. But to be honest, and I don't wanna be harsh here, I'd rather be dumb and care about people with cancer dying than intellectual and indifferent. I guess that makes me really fucking stupid. I guess it does. I guess thinking people shouldn't die is stupid now. I bit my lip politely.

"I mean, if you had it, it would be nice to know, so you could stay home and not infect other people, like old people and people with cancer, huh? Wouldn't it? I mean, I probably didn't have it. But I just kind of think they could've tested me? You know? For other people's sake."

Kristin the German intellectual grinned at me knowingly.

"Jacinta!" she said. "Old people and cancer patients are going to die of the normal flu anyway! They might as well get Corona, it doesn't really make any difference. Did you stock up on toilet paper? I bet you were one of the ones who stocked up on loo roll! So silly!"

"No," I said. "No loo roll. More important things to stock up on, aren't there. Beans. Rice. Asparagus. Garlic and chili oil. That kind of thing."

"I haven't stocked up on anything," the intellectual said.

"I already have all the herbs you need growing on my window sill," the hippy mum said.

"Yeah," I said. "And no nappies either. If we do get Corona, I'm going to do bare-bottom nappy training for two weeks. Might as well put the quarantine to good use."

"You're not going to get it, and even if you do, you're not going to die!" the intellectual said. I nodded.

I can't decide whether German intellectuals really do think that old people and cancer victims dying is literally nothing to worry about – or if they are just pretending that to themselves because they have used up so much panic about eating the brown bits on toast and the deathly *Zug* that will literally kill you and everyone else you know. Maybe they have no energy left to care about Corona.

"Everyone who is panicking about Corona just doesn't realise how many people die of the flu each year," Kristin said happily. I fully imagined her, for a second, turning up to cancer patients' funerals with signs like the Phelps' church people have, but instead of saying "God hates fags" hers would say "YOU WOULD'VE DIED OF FLU ANYWAY YOU FUCKING LOSER".

"It's like Mother Earth is cleaning herself," said Natascha the hippy mum dreamily.

"What?" I said.

"It's like, you know. Detoxing."

"What?," I said.

"Yeah, that's why I am not bothered about the Coronavirus. Because I understand how tired Mother Earth is. She's sending us this virus to clean up a bit. Clean up. You know? We should listen to what she's saying, I think. And instead of working on a vaccine ..."

"We could round up the old and sick and put them in camps, maybe?" I said.

I looked at the two mums I had met at the single mums' breakfast and decided I didn't need any new friends. I have enough totally crazy, slightly fascist friends already, thank you very much.

My son came up to me, gave me a Duplo piece, and shouted "ICE CREAM!" I pretended to lick it and he shouted "NEIN, BESSER ESSEN!" Then he licked it and pushed it into my mouth. "DORBY!" he shouted, which is his word for strawberry. "ESSEN MAMA DORBY ICE CREAM!" His face was covered in snot and I looked at him, and felt very suddenly, and very certainly, that humanity really was doomed.

Chapter Four: D is for ...

Der, die, das:

Der, die, das, die
Den, die, das, die
Des, der, des, der
Dem, der, dem, den
Or, as we say in English:
The, the, the, the
The, the, the, the
The, the, the, the
The, the, the, the

The "the, the, the, the" joke is a cheap one, and it's not even particularly true – at the very least des, der, des, der *should be translated as "of the".*

And still. The sad truth is, you really are going to have to learn these fuckers off by heart. This means that when you learn a new word, you must learn its gender to go with it. There's no getting out of it. Never bother learning to say Brot, *always say* das Brot. *And as for the cases, the terrible truth is – and I am going to tell you the terrible truth – you will probably always get them a little bit wrong. Just as German speakers will never really be able to tell when they should say "I have to" or "I must" or when they say "I've eaten" or "I've been eating", even if you live here in this sad cold city until your dying day you will always sometimes say* dem *and mean* den. *And to be honest, would you really want to be the kind of person who gets them right, anyway? I feel like non-German German speakers who never make these mistakes shouldn't really be trusted. It's not very* sympathisch. *Sort your lives out.*

The der, die, das of It All

I'm sitting with my son, about eight years old, in an Indian restaurant. He wants me to order him a water. He normally drinks *Apfelschorle.*

When the waiter comes, I say "Eine ..." because I am about to say: "Eine Apfelschorle". But then I remember he wants water. So I say: "Eine ... Wasser, bitte."

The waiter walks away, and my son scrunches his eyes up at me disapprovingly. "It's *ein* Wasser, bitte," he says.

"Yeah," I reply. "I know. I know."

He looks at me disbelievingly. "I know!" I say.

"Why do you always get them wrong, then?"

"I don't always get them wrong," I say.

"You can do it in English," he then says, almost forgivingly.

I stare at him in silence for a bit, scrunching my eyes up disapprovingly.

"Erm, Ryan," I say. "What do you mean?"

"In English," he says. "You always get it right in English. A girl. The water. A dog. The football. An apple. I never heard you get it wrong in English."

It's really weird when you're a parent and your kid thinks you're fucking stupid, but the thing is, secretly you think your kid is a bit fucking stupid, too.

"Well, that's because ..." I say slowly. "It's always the same in English?"

Ryan stares at me in silence for a bit, and then a great big smile bursts over his face.

"Yeah!" He shouts. "In English it's always the same. A girl, the girl, a woman, the woman. You don't have this in English!"

I nod.

"THAT'S why it's so hard for you!" he shouts. He laughs a bit. "You can't do this, because it's not like that in English." He shakes his head in amazement.

The popadoms arrive and he is still shaking his head.

"You know, Mum, this whole time, I was thinking you were a bit ... dumb. But it's just your language. Your whole language is dumb, not you!"

I smile at him now.

"Yep," I say. "You're not wrong there."

* * *

Daten: *There are two ways to pronounce* Daten *in German. If you mean, like data and stuff, then it's dar-ten,* daːtn̩. *But if you mean dating someone, then it's dayten:* dɛɪtən̩.

At the moment, there are far fewer words which are spelt the same way but pronounced differently in German than English, but if all this Denglisching keeps on going on as much as it is right now, in a few years' time German spelling will be just as confusing as English.

Dating in Berlin: It's a Shit Sandwich Where the Slices of Bread Are Also Made of Shit, Actually

So, this is what dating in Berlin is like: IT IS REALLY SHIT. IT IS TOTALLY SHIT. IT IS THE SHITTIEST MOST POINTLESS ACTIVITY EVER. It is absolutely, completely, fundamentally and unbearably shit.

You know me, you guys, I love to slag off Germans. Making Germans think I hate them is basically a sexual fetish of mine. "When in doubt, tell Germans they are crap at dancing and racist" is absolutely the motto by which I live my life. I have it written in lipstick on my mirror and everything. But the truth is, dating in Berlin is totally shit whether you are wasting your time with useless German boys or torturing yourself pointlessly with crappy non-German timewasters. It really does NOT matter whether the rubbish boy you date is German or Brazilian, Swedish, US-American, British, South African, whatever. DATING IN BERLIN IS REALLY SHIT. It is the shittiest thing that will ever happen to you. It is fundamentally, deeply, incredibly rubbish.

This is what will happen when you start dating in Germany:

You will be gorgeous, first of all. Maybe you will be a gorgeous German single mother in her early fifties, or maybe you will be a gorgeous Polish single lady in her early twenties. Maybe you will be Indian, Spanish, Greek, Nigerian, I dunno. But you will be GORGEOUS. You will be perfect. You will be a perfect angel. Maybe you won't have that much money, but what you're lacking in money you'll make up for in ambition and drive. Maybe you'll be super-successful in your career though. You might have some mental health issues, but you'll be working on them. And, really, ultimately, you will be PERFECT. You will be GORGEOUS. You will be WONDERFUL. There is literally nothing wrong with any of the women living and working in this town ever, except for the Nazis and women who think Hartz IV people shouldn't get health insurance. Every other woman in Berlin: you are all perfect. I love you all. You are wonderful. You are great, exactly as you are.

And then you will start dating ...

This is what will happen to you: you'll start dating a really, really, REALLY fucking ugly guy – ugly and stupid and boring and POOR. (And I am a socialist. I don't think poor is an insult by the way, I just think if you're rich it kind of maybe makes up for your being ugly, but no, this guy is POOR AS FUCK.) A really, really ugly guy with a silly hat on. He will gladly "agree" to go on a date with you, he might even possibly ask you out himself. This guy will be like, 57 if he's German and still live in a WG, or 27 if he's non-German and not able to speak a word of the language of the country he lives in. THIS GUY IS NOT GOOD ENOUGH FOR YOU. He is so not good enough for you. He isn't even worthy of passing you a glass of water, as the Germans would say. YOU ARE SO OUT OF HIS LEAGUE YOUR LEAGUE TABLE ISN'T EVEN ON THE SAME PAGE OF THE NEWSPAPER. In a normal world – i.e. every city outside of Berlin, nobody would be dating this ugly cunt anyways.

And then what will happen? After your date, maybe straight after your date, maybe he will give you three dates maybe – oh the privilege! – he will even give you three months of his pre-cious life, he will "sadly" tell you that he isn't looking for a girlfriend. He will do this in the manner of a very rich, very wonderful, very generous benefactor giving a poor person the sad news that they can no longer sponsor them through uni. He won't be bitchy about it. He won't be spiteful about it. He will be kind of sad about it.

"I am sorry," he will say. "I don't actually want a girlfriend!"

Oh, for fuck's sake. Fuck me sideways with a toaster, he isn't looking for a girlfriend. THIS IS WHAT DATING IN BERLIN IS LIKE: the ugliest, most boring, stupidest, poorest fuckers aren't "looking for girlfriends" and will inform you of this in these sad, sorry tones like they expect you to die of shock and/or disappointment.

Sometimes he will indulge in super-dickheadish behaviour like stealing money from you, giving you an STI or not telling you about his actual girlfriend, the one he's been going out with/living with for seven hundred years already. (Note: Not dating, because nobody ever dates successfully in this shitty city – they moved here together from Wiesbaden.)

I hate to be a Negative Nancy, but there is literally no point dating in this city. Slim pickings doesn't even begin to cover it. IT'S ANOREXIC PICKINGS HERE. It's bad enough that no Berlin boy is looking for love, ever, it's kind of unbearable that these ugly boring bastards wear their anti-relationshipness on their sleeves like it's some kind of war medal. Not wanting love is a badge of honour in this cold, dark, loveless city. There's no chance of anyone finding love in Berlin. But who needs men anyway, hey girls? The most depressing thing about Berlin is also the most empowering – men don't want girlfriends here, but women, also, once they wake up and smell the ketamine, don't need men. Men. Huh? I wake up every morning and spit on their souls and piss on their corpses. MEN. "Men?" Who needs a man? Didn't you get the memo? A Berlin woman needs a Berlin man like a fish needs an STI. That is, you see, what vibrators and sperm banks were invented for. To make life in Berlin bearable.

* * *

Denglisch: *Denglisch is the word we use for all those English additions to the German language.* Handy *is the most famous one, probably, and* Facility Manager *and* public viewings *are ones that people complain about a lot.*

Most Denglisch is American, huh? It should really be called Damerikanisch. Whack *and* stuff. Cougar. *I learn most American slang from Denglisch, nowadays. British Denglisch is always super old* – Lift. Trampen. Annie-Way *must be the only example of Irish Denglisch? That's exactly what they sounded like. Like Father Ted.* Annie-Way.

Annie-Way! No idea why people stopped saying this. But I guess even Unkraut dies sometimes.

Rollbrett

"There's a new German teacher at school," my son tells me, "who won't let us say skateboard in German class."

"What do you have to say?" I ask.

"*Rollbrett,*" he says.

"*Rollbrett,*" I say, impressed. It sounds really, really, really shit.

Okay, so there are lots of English words in German. People say crazy stuff like *talken* and sometimes they just say, for no reason at all, whole sentences. *I don't get it.* But it's not like there are no German words in English? *Schadenfreude, Zeitgeist, Kindergarten. Umlaut. Verboten.*

This is the difference between English words in German and German words in English: the English people who use the German words don't actually know that the words they are using ARE German. Like my niece, who asked me, a few Christmasses ago, if "verboten" was slang or not.

"You're good at English," she said. "Is verboten slang or is it a real word? Could you write it in an essay?"

"It's slang," I said. "It's German."

"IT'S A GERMAN WORD!" she shrieked. "Yeah, actually, when you see it written down, it does look German. What does it mean in German?"

"Forbidden."

"So what do the Germans say when they want to say verboten?"

This is a good question. The English word *verboten* means something that is just not done, unacceptable, not nice. Like serving champagne in plastic cups or a famous person quote-tweeting someone with 37 followers. Do we have a German word for that? I kind of think we don't – in Germany, things are either *VERBOTEN* or allowed.

The thing I can never imagine happening is an English teacher in Britain making up random English-sounding words to try and stop the kids using German words! We're a long way away from that. Rollbrett.

* * *

Dosen: *Germans call tins or cans of food* Dosen. *Like an American, they can have a* Dose Cola *and a* Dose gebackene Bohnen *(I drink cans of coke and eat tins of baked beans). But they also sometimes have* Büchsen *of sardines. Watch out: Germans HATE HATE HATE tinned food. If you tell them you put tinned beans in a chili con carne, they literally will stop eating it. I don't know what their problem is? They even hate tinned chickpeas, tinned peaches ... even tinned tomatoes. I always wonder, at Aldi and Lidl, who is buying all this tinned stuff. No German I know, anyways.*

Germans Hate Tinned Food – But I Am a Tinfluencer

My German friend Jenni sends me a voice clip over WhatsApp, her voice, soft and gentle, and sad, so sad, her English kind of robotic and American-sounding. (One of the things, by the way, which I have given up for Corona/Quarantine/Quorona-Time/Lent/Christian Ramadan, is trying to force German friends to speak to me in their mother tongue. Whatever, man.)

"I had a hard day today," Jenni says in her soft, robotic voice on the voice clip. "I'm starting to think you might be right about

Drosten. He should probably stick to the lab work more and concentrate less on his podcasts. And he gives a lot of advice which isn't really part of his job, to be honest. It made me feel sad, realising this. Realising I feel this way about him. And the weather outside is beautiful, and I feel so alone. I am alone. I feel so alone. And I am sick, sick, sick to death of canned foods!"

I listen to the voice clip THREE times and feel kind of scared of my own power, like this one time when I was a kid with my Indian granddad in a multi-storey car park and I shouted, as I always did in those car parks: "Drive to the top!" but instead of ignoring me he just said in a happy voice "Okie, dokie" and drove us to the top of the carpark and as we drove up there to the outside world I felt kind of cold inside, powerful and strong but also a bit cold and empty and scared, too.

Jenni thinks I might be right about Drosten! Fucking hell, things are really bad.

Instead of voice-clipping her back, I ring her up.

"Yo Jenni," I say.

"I have to be quiet," she loud-whispers back. "Daisy is asleep in my bed."

"You shouldn't call them canned foods," I say. "Of course canned foods sounds dorky and rubbish." I decide not to mention her 180 degrees horrific U-turn on Drosten, a U-turn so sudden and complete it can be seen from space. "Say tinned food, it sounds much better. Tinned food. Do you want some tinned food? Have you got a tin of sardines? Doesn't that sound fun?"

"No?" she says. "It sounds awful."

"Tinned food is glamorous," I tell her.

"Glamorous?" she says.

"You know what the problem with German people is?" I say.

"We're all Nazis?" she says.

"Well, apart from that," I say cheerfully. "But the biggest problem with German people at the moment is: they haven't noticed how glamorous tinned food is!"

Tinned food is glamorous and if you don't think so, you didn't read enough Enid Blyton growing up. Those sexy midnight feasts after long lacrosse matches – they wouldn't even have happened if tinned food hadn't been invented yet! A delicious glorious fabulous midnight feast – don't invite Gwendolyn or Prudence, they're such sneaks – I'll bring the sausage rolls and the ginger beer and you bring a gorgeous, fabulous, wonderful tin of peaches or pears! And didn't Janet's mother send her a chocolate cake for her birthday?

I am spending my Quorona-Time writing gratitude lists (well, we have to do SOMETHING) and one thing I am grateful for is reading Enid Blyton as a kid. Because I think Enid Blyton is literally the reason I, and millions of other Brits like me, actually prefer the slimy tinned peaches to the boring fresh ones you get at a fruit market (yuck, super-dry).

And now tinned food has come into its own. Tinned food, the glamorous Quorona-survival companion. Now an army of sexy, young, trendy, nutritionally aware preppers know what we need to do: armed only with a few tins, a spice rack, a Jack Monroe cookbook and, of course, our own brilliant imaginations, we can all become tinfluencers! Baked beans (ludicrously expensive in Germany but still gorgeous), mixed with pesto and Worcestershire sauce – YUM YUM YUM! Chickpea and tinned peach curry – I THINK I AM LITERALLY IN HEAVEN RIGHT NOW! Tinned salmon, tinned peas, a ludicrous amount of chilli and pasta bake – DON'T MIND IF I DO! Vegetarian chilli con carne. Tinned mushroom stew. Rice and lentils. Anchovies and rice and lentils. Chilli and cannelloni bean stew. Pasta arrabiata but the tomatoes you use are out of a tin! WHAT'S YOUR FUCKING PROBLEM GERMANY?

Now I don't want to be one of these people nagging everyone to enjoy their Corona Time – or to use it to advance their careers. It's a worldwide pandemic, not a writing and yoga retreat mixed into one. Of course we all have more time right now to work on our writing/yoga skills, but I also think we should be respectful of our dead, and fucking mourn them a bit. I find it a bit grotesque to only want to see the positive things about this time of our history – like at best it is a bit mendacious and at worst it is, and I mean this respectfully, slightly evil. Having said all of that: c'mon Germany! Tinned food is healthy. Tinned food is delicious (if you add spices). Tinned food is cheap. Tinned food is sexy and glamorous. C'mon my darling German babies, channel your inner Enid Blyton, put a pot of tinned beans on, set your spice racks and your imaginations free.

If Dr. Bloody Drosten told you to, you totally would.

Chapter Five: E is for ...

Erziehung: Erziehung *means education, but like in 19th century novels, it's the education parents give their kids. The easiest way of translating is, I guess, parenting –* so Erziehungstipps *becomes parenting advice.*

Nursery school teachers are known as Erzieher, *or* Erzieher*innen, *not* Lehrer or Lehrer*innen. *You only become a teacher if you're teaching actual lessons. A badly raised kid is* schlecht erzogen, *something I accuse my kid of being all the time – it's okay, he gets his own back on me by teaching his little brother "your mum" jokes.*

Bonus trivia: the German supernanny *has renounced the strict* Erziehungstipps *she gave in the early 2000s, and is now in favour of a more loving, flexible, less authoritarian style of* Erziehung.

Confessions of a Permissive Parent

I'm a permissive parent – I think I am, anyway. The signs are there: my oldest boy swears in front of me and even had, aged eleven, a very annoying habit of ending all sentences with the word "bitch," like Jesse from *Breaking Bad*. God, that was embarrassing on the U5, I can tell you. "When we get in, you can do your homework and I'll put dinner on, okay?" My son, cheerfully, in a Jesse from *Breaking Bad* voice: "You bet, bitch!"

My youngest never wears a hat or a scarf. I'm literally so permissive that I don't understand what people mean when they say I should "make" him wear one. WHAT ARE THEY TALKING ABOUT? I try to "make" him wear them, and then three seconds later, he takes them off and throws them off the edge of the Kinderwagen and if I am not paying close attention that's another hat/scarf gone. He wears gloves like 30 per cent of the time, when his hands get cold enough. He actually wears a Corona face mask more willingly than a hat or a scarf – though I think this is because I tricked him into it by telling him only big boys wear masks and babies don't have to. (Although when I say willingly, I mean for like four or five minutes max.)

My friend Tanja is a Tough German Mama. She became a parent for the first time aged 42, grew up in East Berlin, and has lots of dogs.

"Modern German parents!" she says disapprovingly. "They think they should be FRIENDS with their children!"

"Erm," I say politely. "I kind of want to be friends with mine? Is that pathetic of me? Like I want to be their parent and their friend?"

"I am not my child's friend," she replies. "I am their parent, not their friend."

"Yeah, but you don't want to be their enemy either, do you?" I ask.

"No," she says. "I don't see myself as my children's enemy. Of course not! I'm like their dog trainer, to be honest. I raise my kids like I train my dogs. Hard but fair."

"Sounds exhausting," I say. I'm not much of a dog person.

Tough German Mamas like Tanja are always complaining that modern German parents are permissive parents. I remember when Tanja and I were once in a Rewe in Prenzlauer Berg, and a dad asked their kid which flavour yoghurt they liked best, and Tanja whispered to me, really loudly: "That poor child! What a typical modern German parent! That kid is totally overwhelmed with this decision! Just be the parent and choose the yoghurt!"

I whispered back to her: "Maybe he can't decide which yoghurt to get? Maybe he doesn't know?"

Because the thing is, I think Tough German Mamas like Tanja never feel a moment of doubt, ever. Especially not when choosing yoghurt. I think Tough German Mamas like Tanja have never, ever, EVER not known which yoghurt they want to get. I think Tough German Mamas like Tanja would never, ever, EVER feel so indecisive – and indifferent – about which flavour yoghurt they wanted. They would never, like, consult with their kids' preferences before choosing said yoghurt just to make life, you know, a bit easier. Tough German Mamas don't need life to be easy. They kind of want life to be a bit hard.

The Tough German Mamas have it wrong, though. It's not that modern German parents are super-permissive. ALL PARENTS IN BERLIN ARE SUPER-PERMISSIVE. Even the expats. Or do I mean *especially* the expats? Two nights ago, and I blamed Corona for this, but I suspect I was just having fun, my baby and I lay in bed, naked, watching *The Little Mermaid* prequel on Disney+, while eating cold spaghetti I had saved in the fridge. We didn't use forks or anything. I handed him a cold string of spaghetti with my bare hands and he placed it carefully in his mouth with his bare hands and slurped it up. He stayed up until eleven and every now and then we discussed the film together, like stoners.

"Big fish," he said thoughtfully.

"Nice big fish," I said.

"Mermaid one again," he said.

"She's nice, huh," I said.

"Nice mermaid one, dis one," he said, and I handed him

another spaghetti string. He dropped it onto his chest and laughed. I imagined, briefly, what Tough Mama Tanja would say if she could see us now – or even worse, one of the scary Erzieherinnen from the Kita – but I quickly reassured myself that we were only indulging in this sloppy, slovenly, messy cold spaghetti plus *Little Mermaid* gorgeousness because we were working through some distressingly horrendous emotions caused by the Corona crisis.

I know loads of permissive expat parents. Permissive parenting is a Berlin Thing, not a German Thing. I have one American friend who lets her three-year-old pour sugar from the sugar dispenser directly into her mouth at cafés. I have a British friend who lets her seven-year-old order anything he wants to eat from the internet every Sunday. I have a Greek friend who let her kid wear his *Faschingskostüm* to her sister's wedding. It was in a fucking castle and everything and her kid was dressed up like Spiderman.

Here's the thing, though: I am a permissive parent because I am lazy as fuck. It's one of my weaknesses as a person and one of my greatest weaknesses as a parent. I can't be bothered arguing with my oldest boy about his homework and I can't be fucked getting the baby to stop drinking bath water. You know what I did, when the baby started drinking the bath water up like an aquatic ape? I stopped putting bubbles in the bath so the water wouldn't be, like, bad for his stomach, and started putting vitamins in instead.

German Permissive Parents are permissive because they want to make their kids' lives as easy as possible and their own lives almost unbearably hard. Their permissiveness never involves any shortcuts. In fact, some of my German Permissive Parent friends literally wait on their kids HAND AND FOOT AND HEAD AND STOMACH AND NECK TOO.

My friend Lena, who, by the way, can't stand Tanja's guts,

like there is serious beef between them, is telling me about this one time her six-year-old kid Kiera decided to play baby.

"I feel so sorry for Tanja's kids," she says to me bitchily.

"Oh, I know, mate," I reply. "She says she doesn't see herself as their enemy – more like their trainer."

"It's an East thing," Lena says spitefully.

"A dog trainer!" I say.

"So you know when Kiera wanted to be a baby? You know what I let her do? I got out one of her old nappies and let her shit in it."

I stare at Lena in silence for approximately 37 minutes. It's not that I disapprove, exactly. It's more that I can't imagine a world in which I let a toilet-trained kid shit in a nappy just because they're playing baby.

"She needed it," she said. "I'm not her dog trainer. We're collaborating."

German parents never make life easy for themselves, you know. The strict ones treat their kids like dogs and the softies are just absolutely and completely, no pun intended, barking mad. I don't want to sound like some parenting guru or anything, but I think German parents would enjoy parenting a bit more if they realised that you weren't *actually*, actually meant to be perfect. Because nobody's perfect all the time. Not even Germans.

* * *

Einladen: Einladen *means invite, but the thing about inviting people in Germany is it's like how it used to be for posh people in the 70s and 80s in the UK – the person who invites pays. This basically means when someone says to you* "Ich lade dich ein!" *or even, let's be honest "I'm inviting you!" what they really mean is these drinks are on me or "Let me get this."*

Watch out, they don't do rounds over here. I used to find it weird but recently it seems like Anglos are doing rounds less and less too. Also there are just too many Germans who'll order Club Mate or a green tea in a bar to really make rounds a thing.

German Boys: SUDDENLY Really Onboard With Feminism When it Saves Them Money

"We're in Germany, we do things 50/50 here," my good friend, or perhaps acquaintance is a better word here, Sven says, when the cocktail bill arrives.

I look at him in total disgust.

"I'm not one of those feminists who thinks men shouldn't buy women drinks," I say.

"Yes, but we German men are so traumatised by the fierce reaction we get from German women, that we never offer to invite a girl for a drink or for dinner or even a kebab or something."

"I have absolutely no problem with men paying for me," I clarify.

"Yes, but I would not want you to think I am sexist."

"I actually don't think it's sexist," I say. "I actually think it is fair. I am a single fucking mother, the tax system is set up to help men, my German ain't great, I have to do all this unpaid physical labour you know? Get my kid to Kita – I don't get paid for that. Scrub the fucking floors, stay home when he's sick. Why do German women complain so much about the sexism of a man buying you a fucking drink for once in his shitty life, but not about the fact that it is always – and let me repeat ALWAYS – the woman who stays home when a kid gets sick? That like, is literally stealing away my ability to earn money and become more successful in life? But oh, no it's fine, we're all *emanzipiert* now, because we split the bill 50/50?"

"I just, you know," says Sven feebly. "I can't explain it to you. It's how I've been socialised. *Sozialisiert?* Socialised."

"Raised!" I say angrily.

"Not raised?" he says. "There must be a better word. I just couldn't live with myself if I treated you in this disrespectful manner and paid for your drink. I would feel like such a sexist kind of guy, and I'm not you know. I am not sexist. I really respect women as my equals."

"But we're not fucking equal!" I shout at him. "We fucking should be, but we literally are not. German women earn 23 per cent less than German men huh? How much less does a mother earn? The pay gap between mothers and fathers must be even bigger than between men and women! It must be about 50 per cent! There's maternity leave, then you get them into Kita but you have to go and pick the kids up at 4 pm! What can anyone achieve before 3.30pm in the fucking afternoon? Seriously? Do you know how often ..." I glare at Sven angrily, "my ex-husband who was UNEMPLOYED made me call in sick to work to look after our *gemeinsames Kind* even though he had no fucking job and I fucking did because oh, oh, oh, OH, kids need their mums when they're ill. The kid is so fucking *gemeinsam* until it gets sick, then all of a sudden kids needs their mums desperately like you're some kind of fucking Käthe Kollwitz person mixed with Florence Nightingale mixed with Mother Theresa mixed with the mum out of the fucking *Conni* books. Women have to pay, they have to pay, they have to pay for contraception and abortions and childcare, they have to pay with their bodies, with their actual bodies, when they give birth and then afterwards they have to pay with their careers, like you literally have to sacrifice your actual career, your actual success, your actual life, to keep this tiny human being alive and instead of anyone being actually GRATEFUL about it they sneer at you for not being successful enough and ..."

"You don't know how angry German women get when you try to pay for their drinks," Sven says sadly.

It is true, you guys? I am never there when German boys try to pay for women's drinks. I don't know HOW angry they get. All I will say, though, is that it is funny that the one piece of feminism that German boys have taken on 150 per cent, no questions asked, is one that erm, saves them fucking money. The same people who shared that Birgit Kelle piece after *#aufschrei*, who think Alice Schwarzer is ugly and dumb and Anne Wizorek too pretty to be so angry, who don't believe in a women's quota, who think girls are doing too well in school now, who think, in fact, that feminism has gone TOO far in Germany – these same boys would rather die than buy you a fucking drink.

"Anyways, I left my *EC-Karte* at home so you'll just have to pay for me," I tell Sven. Look, I've been living here for nineteen years now. I know *BESCHEID*. The only way to get a German boy to "invite" you is to pretend you left your *EC-Karte* at home and/or say last time you fucked you needed the morning-after pill so they owe you eightteen euros. Be careful though, a lot of them will try to haggle you down to nine. We're in Germany, you know. We do things 50/50 here.

Chapter Six: F is for ...

Fernsehenturm: *So I lived here for a squillion years before I found out it was the* Fernsehturm *and not the* Fernsehenturm. *The TV Tower, not the watching telly tower! (Just think, I used to laugh at my three year old son for calling it the DVD Tower and the whole time I was getting the name wrong myself!)*

Of all the Basic Bitch things you are meant to do with your parents when they come to Berlin, this is the easiest and also the most fun. I mean, to be honest, my parents are happiest of all when I take them to a cheapo Asian restaurant in a shopping centre where the portions are really big and you get free rice or noodles, but the TV Tower is fun, too. Checkpoint Charlie museum is okay, too, all those castles, Schloss Berlin, the colonialist theme park, Schloss Charlottenburg, the DDR Museum, Reichstag, Unter den Linden, and of course, a trip down the Spree. I don't know if your parents are anything like mine, but mine didn't like Potsdam. Not enough cheap Asian places.

Das Boot

It can be a bit embarrassing, sometimes, how obsessed the British are about the Nazis. Obsessed – and kinda fascinated. It can be a bit embarrassing at times.

"Let's do this boat tour thing, Cint," my dad says.

"It's in German," I say, reasonably. "Let's wait for the English language one, it's in an hour."

"Oh, that's okay," my dad says.

"Yeah, we don't mind," my stepmum says.

I stupidly think they mean "that's okay/we don't mind" in the sense of not needing to know what the tour guide says. They, er, don't. They mean "that's okay/we don't mind" in the sense of: you can translate everything he says for us.

Every two minutes one of them asks, really loudly: "What's he say, Cint? Did we bomb that building in the war?"

"Did we bomb that?"

"Why's that building important Cinty? Is it one of the ones we bombed in World War II? Is that what he's saying?"

After about twenty minutes of this, I decide to shout really loudly: "HE ISN'T MENTIONING WHICH BUILDINGS WE BOMBED AND WHICH ONES WE DIDN'T."

My parents are silent for 2.3 seconds, but then my stepmum says, fairly loudly: "We probably bombed all of them and so it's just not worth pointing it out."

Almost as embarrassing as my mother, who, when she visits, insists I ask the waiter at every café we went into if Hitler often came in there to have a cup of coffee.

"Can you ask the waiter, Cint ..." I feel my stomach dropping, "if Hitler ever came in here."

"I'm not asking the waiter if Hitler came in here."

"Well ask him if it was a café during the Nazi times and then we can work it out from there."

"I'm not asking him ..."

"I bet he liked it in here. Kind of posh, isn't it? Where do you think he sat? Maybe the chairs were arranged differently. I don't think he'd sit in the window, do you?"

"He might never have even been inside these four walls."

"Come on, you can practically see the Reichstag from here."

As time goes by, the British fascination with Hitler and the Nazis – especially worse in my parents' generation? – seems more and more bizarre and, I don't know, for want of a better word, creepy. I think what Germans – and also younger generations – can't really imagine is that my parents, who were born in the fifties or the forties, really felt that the Germans, the Nazis, might have won World War II. And so although their giddy excitement about Hitler and the Nazis can seem a bit distasteful to us, for them there was palpable relief involved.

"You'd think they'd have changed the U-Bahn announcement since the Nazi times," my mum said, the first time she ever visited me. We were on the U1 and the recorded U-Bahn guy had just barked "Zurückbleiben bitte!" and my mum's voice was embarrassingly loud.

"I think they probably have?" I whispered back.

"They most definitely haven't!" My mum said back. "Zurückbleiben bitte!"

But sometimes, to be quite honest, with all the Brexit bollocks and the D-Day nostalgia, it can feel like it's the Brits who stayed back – or, even, perhaps, fell behind.

* * *

Ficktermin: Fick *means fuck, and* Termin *means appointment, and* Ficktermin *means fuck date. But beware: it's a made-up word. I made it up myself, in my head, out of my own imagination. Still, I think the whole point of being able to speak German is the ability to make up composite nouns as you see fit. As soon as you put two German words together, they always sound kind of real.* Spieltermin. Hausmaus. Lieferdienst. Ersatzspatel. *I could literally do this for hours. It's my* Sprachhobby.

My Friend Lola

My little friend Lola phones me up. Lola is so young, so tiny, so little, such a tiny, little millennial pixie, that any time she phones me up on the actual telephone, I think it must be an emergency. Like, basically, if she rings me up, I think someone has died.

"Lola!" I gasp into my WhatsApp. "ARE YOU OKAY?"

"No, Jacinta!" she wails desperately at me. "I just found out *Ficktermin* isn't a proper word!"

"Oh," I say.

"I thought it was an actual word!"

"No," I say guiltily. "I just made it up, like a funny German version of fuck date?"

"Oh my god, Jacinta, you're not allowed to INVENT words like that!"

"I think you are, actually," I say calmly.

"This is why German men think I am such a slut!" she says.

"Well, that's not the only reason," I say diplomatically. "Lola, are Ficktermine even allowed right now?"

"Oh yeah sure," she says breezily. "Totally legal. Just not allowed to invite people from, like, seven different households."

"Okay," I say. "Well, good luck!"

Chapter Seven: G is for ...

Gendern: *German is a much more gendered language than English, at least. Most nouns used to describe a person have a male form:* der Lehrer, *a female form:* die Lehrerin, *a male plural:* die Lehrer, *and a female plural:* die Lehrerinnen.

Now, the problem is that there are male and female teachers and so really you need a plural for both. For years, people said die Lehrer *and meant* Lehrer *and* Lehrerinnen. *Fairly sexist people (no offence you guys) want to continue doing so, and to be quite honest, a LOT of people, when talking, still do so. Quite feminist people either say* Lehrerinnen und Lehrer *(bit of a mouthful, you have to admit) or* Lehrer*innen *or* Lehrer:innen. *An almost imperceivable glottal stop is used to express the star or the colon.*

Germans love their language, and they weirdly haven't noticed how ugly it is, and so a lot of fairly sexist people think stars and colons are too ugly and yucky for words. There are other solutions – Lehrende *or* Lehrkäfte *for example.*

It's kind of hard for English speakers to give a shit. We try to, honest we do, and if I had to, I'd join Team *innen *every time, but it is hard for us to understand, mainly because the -er ending in English is gender neutral already and so you can't help thinking chill out, guys, why don't you just pretend* die Lehrer *means* die Lehrer*innen *and it's all good? However, over the years I've come round to thinking this isn't the perfect solution, mainly because alt-*

hough a female teacher in the singular can be a teacher, a Lehrerin *isn't a* Lehrer. *In fact, I've become so used to the German way of thinking that I actually think the word tennis player is excluding female tennis players a tiny bit – not as much as the German word* Spieler *does – Serena Williams could be the best tennis player in the world, but she'll always be the best* Spielerin.

I sometimes wonder if the English language might get influenced by all this German gendering and start bringing back our female nouns. We do still say actress and stewardess and waitress – such traditionally feminine jobs that the -ess versions sounded like words in their own right, and not female equivalents of male jobs – but wouldn't it be kind of sexy and glamorous if we started saying authoress and poetess and murderess again? Murderess is especially sexy, I think: a murderous murderess. Female murderer just doesn't have the same ring to it?

The weirdest thing about the whole gender thing is that in German, the slightly sexist people want to call female teachers Lehrer, *whereas in English, it's the other way round, with the slightly sexist people wanting to call Angelina Jolie an actress and not an actor.*

German Husbands: Getting Jealous of People's Cousins Since 2004

I have a German-Russian friend who really hates all my Russian-Russian friends, I don't really get it, but it reminds me of how you will get Scottish people together and think they'll really get on, because they seem like, exactly the same person to you, but because one of them is Protestant and one of them is Catholic they spend the whole night sniping at each other like enemies. I don't get it, I love everyone from the East London/Essex area. Although actually, yeah, when there's a load of lads on a stag do on the U-Bahn, I pretend not to speak English. Maybe I do get it.

But now I have finally united the divided forever: my German-Russian friend and Russian-Russian friend, both married to German-German men, are ganging up on me about the English language.

"Maybe English men are less jealous than German men?" the German-Russian says.

"A lot less jealous!" the Russian-Russian says.

"What do your husbands say? What do your boyfriends say? A German boyfriend wouldn't like it. And a German husband would divorce you! He would say, here you go, you slut, I give you a divorce, see how you like this. My boss says I have to stay later tonight. I'm going to see a neighbour. I'm having coffee with my cousin. German men. Get Jealous. Very, very jealous."

"Of COUSINS?" I yelp. I always considered German men kind of like too indifferent and meek to get really jealous. I always thought they were kind of ... too lazy to get jealous.

The thing is, actually, I'm so German now that when I speak English, I have to specify everyone's gender. My anecdotes go like this: "So my female colleague said her male neighbour thinks his female cousin's male boss is fucking the female CEO ..."

Still though! COUSINS. Nothing to be jealous of in this day and age.

"You have to be a bit paranoid to be jealous of a cousin," I say.

My German-Russian friend shrugs and then sighs, slightly smugly.

"Some of my male cousins," she says knowingly, "are very attractive."

Chapter Eight: H is for …

Handy: *A very handy word for mobile telephone, I am sure you'll agree!*

Fake Denglisch

Germans are always complaining about Denglisch, and you can't really blame them, can you? Sometimes I think that by 2030 there'll be no nouns and hardly any verbs left in the German language. It'll be all, like: "Also, ich wollte ins Shopping Center goen aber ich hatte keine Time in der End also deswegen ging ich doch schnell in die Pharmacy." SORRY – I kind of thought that was going to turn out funnier than it did. Sorry. Actually that's just blatantly how everyone is going to talk in 2030.

So, Germans complain a LOT about Denglisch and stuff – but it's kind of like how people complain about parents being on their phones too much at the playground – it's something to complain about but nobody, literally nobody, cares enough to change their own behaviour. Also, I do think they complain about Denglish a tiny, tiny bit too much? It's not like there's no German words in English, is it now?

Some German words are so *eingeenglischt*, you don't even know they are German anymore – *hamster*, for example – and some are barely even *eingeenglischt* at all, but you would never, ever, ever need to translate them – *Kindergarten, Autobahn, Hausfrau.*

ALSO: some of the words us Anglos get the blame for aren't even English at all! Take *Handy* for example. *Handy* is a Japanese anglicism. It's not really Denglisch. It's Djapanisch!

Young people in Britain know what a Handy is, too.

"Oh, I forgot my Handy at home!" I said at my granddad's funeral.

"You forgot your WHAT?" exclaimed my aunt, in a slight state of panic.

"Is that the German word for mobile telephone?" asked another, slightly younger aunt, vaguely.

"Yeah!" A twenty-year-old cousin said. "Love that word! Handy. Where is my Handy? I need to phone someone with my Handy. It's very handy. Jaaaaaaa ..."

You can hate Denglisch all you want, and most people do, but you'd have to have a heart of stone not to admit that Handy is a very, very handy word. There's a reason why no English speaker lives here for longer than five days without picking up this word and using it forever. The reason is that telephone, phone, mobile and cell are all TOTALLY SHIT WORDS. Maybe it's too simplistic to say that the beautiful Proper German language is being brutally vandalised and defiled by the ugly, hungry, capitalistic English tongue. The truth is: the Japanese invented it, the Germans embraced it and now the Anglos are delighted by it. Wo ist mein Handy?

* * *

Hartz IV: *Pronounced, somewhat aptly, "heart's fear" this is what German welfare, or* Arbeitslosengeld II, *is called. The guy who introduced it to the country was called something Hartz – probably*

Robert or Andreas, let's face it – or maybe even Peter – and got involved in a really saucy sex worker scandal a few years later. Posh Germans think it is the most generous welfare system known to man, but the truth is, while it is more generous than the American system, it can be really punitive and it isn't enough to live on, especially if you have kids.

Heart's Fear

"I never ate so well as I did the summer I was on Hartz IV!" my German friend Leonie announces, as she gets our Sunday buffet brunch ready. There's sun-dried tomatoes and organic hummus and organic guacamole and Dinkel cookies and plates and plates of French cheeses and weird salami and goat's cheese and olives and a really weird type of mustard and also scones and a walnut and pumpkin pie baking in the oven.

"Really?" I ask sceptically.

Rich white Germans are forever telling me how well they ate the "summer" they were on Hartz IV. It's weird because I went on Hartz IV for lockdown times and we ate okay-ish. And I was always earning the maximum amount of extra money you were allowed to earn. And it was like ... okay. ISH. With an emphasis on the ish. In fact, I did a petition to try and get Hartz IV parents food vouchers or maybe even food parcels, to try and make up for the school meals their kids were missing, which some people said was poor-shaming because actually you should just let poor people decide what they wanted to spend their money on. Maybe people are right, maybe it was a bit poor-shaming. But no Hartz IV mums thought that it was. They all just thought we should get food vouchers or food parcels to help us through lockdown. One person even sent me an e-book full of Hartz IV-friendly recipes which was full of really quite okay recipes – stuff like get a carrot, fry it in vegetable oil with some garlic – mix in some rice. It's a nice idea, huh? But I dunno. You can't eat that every day of the week. Carrot rice, I dunno ... I mean, they're right. Carrot rice, it's healthy, it's filling. But still. Nobody, especially not a teenager, can live off carrot rice alone and people who think it's easy – or possible, even – to keep a teenager and a toddler both healthy AND full on Hartz IV have never met a teenager or a toddler, I don't think.

Leonie tops up the rioja in my glass and asks me if I want to try my next coffee with a new kind of almond milk she discovered, which actually isn't environmentally unfriendly.

"Yeah!" I say.

I wonder if all the posh Germans who "ate so well" the summer they were on Hartz IV are just lying to themselves, or if doing it for a summer is easier than doing it for years and years and years. If you go on Hartz IV for the summer, you don't need winter boots do you?

"Try this," Leonie says, and brings me a vegan Flammkuchen.

I wolf it down, it's truly delicious.

"Did you really eat well, the summer you were on Hartz IV?" I ask her.

"Oh yeah," she says. "The thing is, Jacinta, I'm a really good shoplifter, you know."

* * *

Hund: Hund *is a dog,* Hündin *is a bitch, but not in a bad way,* Dogge *is a big dog, like a bull dog and* Wauwau *is what kiddies say for doggie. My kid once got corrected by a punk begging for money for weed on the floor for calling his dog a* Wauwau: *"Das ist kein Wauwau, das ist ein Hund!"*

I've always thought those people who really love their pets are slightly mad – all that money, all that effort, all that mouth-kissing – but NOBODY is crazier than a Berliner single mum who adopted a pug during lockdown.

"Please cuddle Ophelia," my friend Marisa whispers melodramatically to me at the park. "I really want you two to like each other." She promptly hands me something that looks like a slightly obese guinea pig, only it has been wiggled into a dog collar. The dog blinks at me. She slobbers. I hand her back to Marisa as soon as possible. I don't want to get dog slobber on me.

"Are you sure this is a real dog?" I ask politely. "She seems a tiny bit ... rodent?"

"She's a total princess," Marisa says happily. "You can kiss her on the mouth if you want to. She doesn't have Corona. Probably."

As I politely decline, Ophelia looks at me: bemused, indifferent, superior. She really is super sweet, in a snobby, slightly obese guinea pig kind of way.

"Anyway, I've made you godmother," Marisa announces airily.

"Don't people normally have to consent to becoming pugs' godmothers?" I ask.

"It's a real honour for you, actually," she explains. "Ophelia only has, like, twenty other godparents. And it'll do your kids good, hanging out with her. My sociopathic kids are, like, 27 per cent less sociopathic now they have a dog to look after. And plus, if you kiss her on the mouth it's really good for your immune system. Look, let me show you."

AAARGH! So now, I, Jacinta Nandi – someone who hates dogs (with their disgusting dog poo which will probably make your kid go blind) even more than she hates cats (I dunno, I just hate them) – have accidentally become a pug godmother. Some people achieve pug godmother status, others have it thrust upon them in the park.

I officially HATE dogs. I hate the *Kampfhund* ones, and find the little, yappy ones annoying. I hate the way they whine at you and bark and then, if you're on your period, they start humping your leg and sniffing your *Muschi*.

AND NOW THE ENTIRE CITY ADOPTED A DOG OVER LOCKDOWN. Like, is there anyone left in Berlin without a dog? My friend Simon broke lockdown rules and went to Poland to adopt a half-wolf. My friend Tanja got herself a *Mischling* from the *Tierheim*. And all the single mums bought pugs or some genetically modified monstrosity with a weird oversized head wobbling away on its tiny body.

What I hate about dogs more than all the shit and the barking is all the fuss. WHY DO BERLINERS LOVE DOGS SO MUCH? Berlin, a city that is so unfriendly you get confused when people from out-of-town ask you what your next-door neighbour's name is (WHY WOULD I KNOW THAT? I'M NOT PSYCHIC), is also a city that loves dogs as much as it hates babies.

Have you ever gone to a party with a baby? People act like you're just doing it to spite them. But turn up with a dog and it's FIIIIIINE. The most unbearably trendy hipsters and ridiculously hard punks are cooing and gushing and swooning and basically orgasming – you even see posh people getting down on all fours to join in the doggy mayhem like they're the canine version of Mowgli.

The only people who know their neighbours are dog owners. Sparking up conversation in the park with a stranger is almost impossible – unless you have a furry friend with you, trying to lick said stranger's own furry friend's arsehole out.

Some Germans don't even *know* you're actually allowed to talk to anyone you meet, even if they're not a relative. But it is exactly these people who will stop on the street to chat with fellow dog walkers and have those ridiculous doggie conversations. I don't know what they talk about, I kind of zone out: dog names, age, diet, expensive operations, the best vet in town, allergies. I don't actually think mums in Berlin are helicopter parents – but I know a few helicopter dog owners.

Oh well, if you can't beat them, join them, as the saying goes. I'll be at the dog park with my darling godchild this weekend. If you see me, come over and say hi. Mouth-kissing with the pug is optional.

Chapter Nine:

I is for …

Impfen: *The boring thing about Corona is the way it split the country. It's been like a German Brexit. People seem to be either vaxxed or anti-vaxxers here. It's boring and depressing, and while I wish everyone would get vaxxed, I hate the whole debate.*

Impfen *is the German word for vaccinate – a lot of expats write it in English: Are you impfed? Some of them even change the f to a cheeky ph "I haven't managed to get the five year old imphed yet!"*

Geimpft = *vaccinated*

Ungeimpft = *unvaccinated*

Impfgegner*innen = *anti-vaxxers*

Impfpflicht = *vaccine mandate, a great word because of the "pfpf". If they ever do introduce a vaccine mandate, I want to sell Karl Lauterbach the slogan* "Impfpflicht am Ende des Tunnels" *and become a millionaire.*

The Kind of Women Who Are Anti-Vaxxers in Berlin Are Kind of Surprising TBH

It always surprises me what kind of women are anti-vaxxers in Berlin. When I think of Anglo anti-vaxxers, I think of real hippies, total Christians or, to be frank, almost-Nazis. But the kind of Berlin mothers who will come out with anti-vax stuff often seem to be slightly too "normal" or "intelligent" to be this sceptical about one of humanity's greatest achievements. Or maybe just too cool? I feel like you can be quite cool here – and still be a bit of an *Impfgegner*.

"You know people think all anti-vaxxers are dumb and ignorant," says my friend Kristin. Nice, funky, cool, feminist, NORMAL German Kristin. Cool. Kristin is cool. I know she's cool. She has cool hair, and a kind of silvery blue fringe. She's cool. She's my cool friend Kristin.

"Yeah," I say. "I don't think they're dumb. I just think they're wrong and confused. I actually think one of the reasons we should introduce mandatory vaccinations is literally just because having the choice is too confusing for people. Sometimes I wonder whether humans can really cope with choice? Like, maybe if we had the option of not wearing a seatbelt there would be all these theories about how it's bad for your neck and stuff? But I realise I sound a tiny bit Soviet-y right now."

"Oh, they can't introduce an *Impfpflicht* in Germany," Kristin says cheerfully. "Because of all the Stasi stuff, you know?"

I find it weird that Germans can get over their *Stasi-Vergangenheit* enough to have a weird *Meldepflicht*, (which, by the way, in my entire twenty years in this country I have never been able to get my mother to understand, she STILL thinks it is a police database of paedophiles and sexual deviants) or a *Schulpflicht*, which, like you know, seems pretty illegal to everyone who doesn't live in Germany (people think we have compulsory schooling in other countries, but in most other countries homeschooling, as in parent-led education, is an optional form of education. In Germany it not only isn't, but school starts literally in the middle of the night (8 am) and you're not allowed to miss one day of term-time. ... But mandatory vaccinations is a step too far. I actually think the police knowing where everyone in the fucking country lives is creepy as fuck, and the state forcing us to send our kids into schools is authoritarian as hell, but a little needle in your skin for a couple of seconds for the good of the whole society is, I dunno, kind of a *Pipifax* to me. But what do I know? I guess it is a legacy of the Stasi times, huh? Without wanting to sound too flippant, all those sterilised athletes and that, people are a bit traumatised?

"I suppose they can't," I say.

"People say *Impfgegner* like it's such an insult. *Impfgegner*. Like it's such a dehumanising word."

"Yeah," I say. "I suppose it is."

"I am not an *Impfgegner*," she says.

"Of course you're not!" I say. I know she isn't, her haircut is too funky and cool. Blue fringe and that.

"I'm an *Impfquestioner*," she says.

I stare at her. Maybe her hair is not quite as funky and cool as I think it is. I stare at her blue fringe and it gets dorkier by the second.

"An *Impfquestioner*?" I say.

"You'd have to be stupid not to question why the government's wanting to inject your kids, wouldn't you?"

"It's. Erm. So they don't get measles?" I say politely. Her fringe isn't ironic, I decide. I thought it was an ironic fringe. It was never ironic.

"Of course I immunise my kids," she says. "But I just do a different schedule than the state wants me to."

"Oh," I say, gulping.

"And the measles one, for example," she says brightly, "is not on my schedule. Not for the," nice long pause, "foreseeable future."

FUCKING HELL I AM FRIENDS WITH AN IMPFGEGNERIN!

There have been a lot of debates recently, on Facebook, for example, about whether, when we finally get a Corona vaccine

(DR. DROSTEN WE BELIEVE IN YOU 100 per cent!), there will need to be an Impfpflicht. Various people, some of them Nazis, believe weird things about Bill Gates, things which kind of bore me, to be honest.

There are conspiracy theories I kind of "like" about Corona. It was invented by China because they knew the Chinese were more obedient than Westerners and so more Westerners would die and they could take over the world! It was a cure for HIV that got out of hand! It is a biological weapon which attacks the organs of people of colour! That kind of thing. But the Bill Gates stuff bores me. So there are a few people who claim that when we finally do get a vaccine, there will be mandatory vaccinations all over the world and everyone will get injected by this Bill Gatesy substance. But there are also some Berliners, really non-Nazi people, who think that when we do finally get this vaccine made, because of mums like Kristin, we will need an Impfpflicht.

What do you guys think? Maybe I am being super un-German here, but I don't really understand why Schulpflicht and Meldepflicht are okay, but an Impfpflicht or a Maskenpflicht, which may save so many lives, totally Stasi. But maybe we won't need mandatory vaccinations, anyways?

This is what my solution would be: Germany should act like there's an Impfpflicht for the Coronavirus vaccine, but it won't actually be an actual Pflicht. We won't go to our own personal doctors in our own personal, intimate doctor's practice with our own little AOK cards and sit down and having a nice chat about if we feel like getting immunised against Corona or not.

We will not be writing about our Corona vaccinations in our stupid yellow Impfpasses (which are the smallest things ever made into official documents ever). We won't be talking about it as if it's a choice. Instead, the Gesundheitsamt will write to everyone in the Bezirk, demanding they come in and get the lovely jab. And if you don't go, you get a warning. And if you don't go then, you get a really STERN warning. But maybe – just maybe – if we do things this way, you won't actually need a hefty fine for ignoring the warnings because enough people will do what they're told to protect us anyway.

What do you guys think? Have you ever been surprised to discover an otherwise very clever and cool seeming German is a secret anti-vaxxer? And will mandatory vaccinations be our only way out of this Corona nightmare?

"Don't you think," I say quietly, "that you maybe have a responsibility towards, like, other people? To get vaccinated?"

"You can't live your life like that," Kristin says.

"Can't you?" I ask.

"You can't live your life in fear," she says.

"I think it's okay," I say, "to be scared of dying. Or maybe killing others. I think that's an okay thing to be scared of."

"Yes, but where will it end?" she asks.

I suddenly see where it's going to end. An Impfpflicht. I hope we don't have to do one – but I think we will.

* * *

Indianer: Indianer *or* Indianerin *means Indian, but not in an Indian-Indian way. In an American Indian, or Native American way. (A more PC term would be* amerikanische Ureinwohner*).*

If someone comes from India, they are an Inder *or an* Inderin, *if they're female. I really confused people when I first arrived here, and told them all: "Mein Papa ist ein Indianer."*

Btw, the word Asian, asiatisch, *is used in the American English way, not the British English way. If you're British Asian, it's best to say* Brite/Britin mit indischen/pakistanischen/chinesischen/bangladeshi Wurzeln. *There is also no good word for non-white,*

I often just say nicht-weiß, *but sometimes I say PoC. Black people are* Schwarze *but if they have African roots, you can totally say* Afrodeutsche.

Innocence

White Germans are so clueless on race, it's almost like you can't hate on them for it (I SAID ALMOST, GUYS!). They are literally all like this clueless naïve granny who vaguely knows racism is bad and generally thinks she should use the correct words to describe people – but is also way too proud of herself for caring.

My German friend Jana, after I sleep over at her place, invites me to come over to a super posh *Kindergeburtstag* – kids' birthday party – some people from her Kita are having.

"They're so rich," she says. "They won't mind you tagging along too."

These are Prenzlauer Berg parents: the dad's a filmmaker, the mum is an ex-model-turned-yoga teacher, they live in this two-story luxury apartment where apparently the top floor is like an Instagram loft palace and the bottom floor is a kid-friendly family flat. Jana makes out like the kids are allowed – or even encouraged – to smear paint and glue and glitter glue and mud and snot all over the walls.

They literally sound like the coolest, poshest, poshest, coolest couple in Berlin.

"I saw she has a selfie of herself with Heidi Klum on her Facebook," Jana says.

"Wow," I say, genuinely impressed.

"So this kids' birthday party is, like, Cowboys and Indians theme," Jana says, nonchalantly.

"WHAT!" I exclaim.

"It's just a kid's birthday party," she says.

"What is this, 1976?" I say.

"It's not racist," she says.

"I didn't say it was racist," I say.

"You were thinking it. You English speakers are always nagging us about racism."

"1972, actually. There were even people in 1976 who would've been embarrassed to go to a Cowboys and Indians themed party."

"The thing is," she says, "we Germans never actually killed any American Indians."

"This is true," I say encouragingly. "Well done!"

"I suppose you are too principled to come?" she asks.

"Erm," I say. The truth is, I want to check it out. I always thought the German fascination with Native Americans was a dorky East German thing (I also always thought, by the way, that the dorky East German fascination with line dancing came about because line dancing had been banned in the East Times by the Stasi, but it turns out, apparently, THAT THEY ACTUALLY JUST REALLY LIKE IT) but enough West Germans have told me that they too love all the *Winnetou* stuff for me to realise I can't blame the DDR for this one.

So we go with Jana to the incredibly posh Prenzlauer Berg Kindergeburtstag. I don't get to see upstairs, but the downstairs flat seems posh enough for me. I get talking to a photographer who actually grew up in Prenzlauer Berg. He tells me he rents his flat for like 500 euros or something, I nearly die of jealousy, Jana starts taking photos of everyone.

"Don't put my photo on Facebook, Jana!" I call warningly.

The East Berlin photographer approves.

"Very good," he says. "You need to protect yourself from Facebook."

"Oh it's not that," I say. "But imagine what American friends would say if they saw these photos!"

"What?" he asks, confused.

"Well, imagine what they'd think!" I say.

"What would they think?" he asks.

"Well," I say. "I think they'd think it was a bit racist."

Total blankness.

"Racist?"

"Well, you know?" I say. "All the cowboys and Indians running around?"

"Why would Americans think it was racist?"

"Well, you know ..." I feel a bit guilty for telling him the truth. "American people are more likely to know Native Americans, right? They maybe even went to school with them and stuff. For them it's not just a costume, like dressing up like a Viking or a pirate. I guess you'd feel differently about this party if you knew some Native Americans."

"But why would Native Americans think it was racist?" he asks.

He looks so totally clueless. My kid runs past, a box of face paints in his hand. Rich people's kids' birthday parties can get totally out of hand sometimes. I'm getting out of here before the blackfacing starts, I decide.

"Just a bit disrespectful," I say.

"For us in Germany," he explains, "the cowboys are the baddies. And the Indians are the goodies! None of this is racism. This isn't racism! It's admiration."

I nod politely. Totally clueless, I think. They should just stick to making good bread and never speak again.

* * *

Integration: Integration *means integration,* integriert *means integrated. When I first arrived in Germany, I had never heard Brits talking about integrated people before. I translated it in my head as "Westernised", which was a kind of insult among British Asians for people who had lost their roots. It's a sign of how boring and basic and depressing humanity is that now the Brits are now also always (ALWAYS) going on about how integrated or unintegrated various people are, yawn.*

Integration

I have lived in Germany for twenty years, and I have never been able to work out what White Germans mean when they go on about integration. What are they literally talking about? Is it having a nice job? Loads of 26-year-olds from Brooklyn who work from home and don't speak a word of German earn shitloads more money than the average German, though. Is it speaking the language well? It's really fucking hard though, the only non-native speakers who speak it well are literally spies and stuff. Eating pork every day? But does that mean German vegans aren't integrated? Watching German telly? You're just being weird now.

Back in the olden days, i.e. before 2015, right, and the *sogenannte Flüchtlingskrise* (the racistly named "refugee crisis"), I used to rant lots about how an English expat who liked going to the English theatre to watch plays in English was considered "integrated" whereas Turkish people who watched Turkish soap operas or films on Sky were considered a total blight on German society. But the popularity of Netflix, Amazon, Disney Plus and also all the refugees who came in 2015 learning German so fucking quickly mean that this point seems totally unoriginal now. To be honest, most German people I know aren't "integrated" either – they just speak German quite well because they were born here and that's literally it.

All this talk about *Integration* is just a racist dog-whistle which places the blame for racism, at a structural and personal level, with the victims. That's all. Human beings are the same everywhere. People do things they like doing, they eat things they like eating, they go to shops they like shopping in, and they watch TV shows they find interesting. People are human, and they make mistakes, and it's hard to be poor, and integration doesn't exist. I know it doesn't exist, because people keep telling me how well integrated I am and I still drink tea with milk in it. So there.

Chapter Ten: J is for ...

Jugendamt: *I haven't talked about* Amts *much yet! Or, as we say in German,* Ämter. *(German plurals are, by the way, a fucking nightmare, your best bet is to just randomly throw umlauts around and add either an R or an N on the end and hope for the best.**) In Germany, it can sometimes seem like there is an* Amt *– an official office – for everything. There's the* Postamt, *the post office, which isn't an official* Amt *anymore. There's the* Arbeitsamt *– the job centre, basically. The* Wohnungsamt *– the housing office. There's the* Meldeamt, *which is where you register your address in Germany, the* Finanzamt, *yuck, the tax office, the* Gesundheitsamt, *which, apparently, you can go to if you want to get the cost of your birth control pills reimbursed, or a man to check your kid's liced up hair for you – and the* Jugendamt.

The Jugendamt *is hard to translate. Youth social services? Social services? Youth welfare office? They do a lot of things that the social services in Britain, or child protection in the States, do. You know, check we're not all abusing our kids and stuff. But they do more boring things than that, too. They pay money for people whose exes are too poor to pay child support – this department is the*

* For that reason Jacinta asked me to correct some plurals in this book. So I will. By the way, the (very rare) German plural of "Plural" ist "Plurale", no R, no N. – just saying. — German editor

Unterhaltsvorschusskasse – *and they give you certificates to help you pay your childcare costs – and they might even help you with therapy costs, too.*

Without wanting to get into too much detail, I think Jugendamt *was the word my mum got to know the best over the course of my twenty years in Germany. She used to spell it* Yukhindamft. *"How did the meeting at the Yukhindamft go?"*

Unterhaltsvorschusskasse

The people who work at the Amts – or the *Ämter* – are called *Beamte* which I always think sounds like a really boring 50-year-old German woman's name. Like: Brigitte, Beate, Renate, Beamte. Which is apt, because these are the ladies who work at the Amts.

People translate *Beamte* as civil servant, but when I hear the word civil servant I always think of people who work at Downing Street, or in Whitehall, losing important documents on the bus and stuff. Beamtes are a bit more boring than that. They're just the ladies who work at the Amts.

The ladies who work at the Amts are, and I mean this in a really respectful way, total fucking bitches. You have one piece of paper missing – a piece of paper which maybe, like, doesn't fucking exist because you weren't born in this fucked-up, heartless country run by fucked-up, heartless robots – and their eyes close, like you see these shutters going down, and they glaze over and close up and their hearts are walled in and there is literally no point speaking to them anymore. They're not human anymore. There's nothing there. They're like fucking Daleks, seriously.

I once got my ex husband to sign a *Vollmacht*, but for various annoying reasons he refused to sign the official Vollmacht form, but scribbled a message of his own on the back of the paper, and the lady at the Amt held it up like it was toxic waste and whispered at me contemptuously: "This is not a Voll. Macht. Do you understand what a Voll. Macht is? VOLL. MACHT. This is not *voll*!"

(By the way the word *Vollmacht* means complete power, or, if you are not a sociopath, permission slip.)

They're just awful human beings and the world would be better if they were all fired or sent into early retirement and replaced by migrants on temporary contracts who actually smiled at you and did their job and stuff. This is the most neoliberal thing I think and you won't change my mind on the matter, sorry. I'd fill the Meldeamt and the Standesamt and the Gesundheitsamt with 26-year-old Polish people with nice teeth, great German, fantastic English and an actual fucking desire to be there. Fire the Beamtes, it's time for the Agnieszkas to take over.

If you ever do meet a human Beamte, you have to take advantage of it though. I met a human one once, at the Meldeamt. I didn't have the correct piece of paper, I think it was also a Vollmacht, and just at the very second she was about to notice, I started telling her that my dad was born in India, but came to England in the late fifties, and was the first "black" kid at my junior school, and back in those days they called Indians black. She literally got so interested in my story she just sat there, totally fascinated, and melded me unvollmachted as fuck an.

Also there are two really happy Amts in Germany, and I've been to both of them. The first is the place where you get freed/liberated/*befreit* (it seems a bit weird to call it liberated in English, but seriously the people do seem so free afterwards) from their church tax. They bounce out of that room, like ten kilos lighter. The second happy Amt is the *Unterhaltsvorschusskasse.*

The Beamtes who work in this Amt are still totally Beamte-types, but tough as nails and they hate men. They hate men so much. I MEAN THEY THINK MEN ARE SHIT. The Beamtes at the Unterhaltsvorschusskasse are like feminist cops who've seen loads of dead prostitutes and so now hate men, but not in a woke way. And these ladies are more likely to have red hair than blonde hair. They're the coolest Beamtes in town

"Has he ever given you any money?" the Unterhaltsvorschusskasse lady asks me.

I scoff.

"No," I say scornfully.

"Men!" she says contemptuously.

"What are they good for?" her colleague says disdainfully.

My boy starts running around her office and I try to get him to stop.

"Can you get him to stop?" she asks me.

"He's a bit bored," I say apologetically.

"Does he take after his dad?" she asks and we all laugh together maliciously.

"You've got his birthdate wrong here," she says. I stare at the form. God what kind of mum am I? I got his BIRTHDATE wrong at the Jugendamt. For fuck's sake.

"That's his due date!" I say. "I'm not a Rabenmutter. I just forgot and wrote his due date instead of his real birthdate. I'm not a bad mum."

"We at the Unterhaltsvorschusskasse don't care if you're a good mum or not," she says. "That's our colleagues down the corridor. All we want is that you get your money."

"That's all we care about," her colleague says. "Money, money, money."

"But for what it's worth, I don't think you're a Rabenmutter at all," my lady says. "If you were a Rabenmutter, your kid would be a bit more scared of you! He'd be better behaved! Get out of here, I can't work with all this noise and chaos around me."

It's probably just about the nicest thing a German Beamte ever said to me.

Chapter Eleven: K is for …

Kaltmiete: *Your* Kaltmiete *is your basic rent – like, literally what it costs to rent the actual apartment you live in. Despite living here for a squillion years, I've never really understood what the point of knowing this figure is – because the* Warmmiete *is what you end up paying anyway, once you've added in heating costs.*

Back in the Olden Days, aka the year 2000, when I arrived in Germany, I thought all the flats in Zitty *described as* Kaltmiete *didn't have any heating. I don't mean only had* Ofenheizung *– a big oven in the living room instead of central heating, which was really common back then, and still not completely, completely unheard of now, though getting rarer and rarer by the second – I literally just thought toughed out the winters, putting extra jumpers on, shivering under blankets. I mean, Germans seem tough, right? This seemed plausible to me. I guess I must have asked someone what it meant and they said* "ohne Heizung" *and I thought they literally meant WITH NO HEATING and brrrrrrr, brrrrr, brrrrrrr.*

Young people I tell this story to ask me why I didn't just google the answer, but I don't think I knew about Google back then. So I just wandered through the city, ringing up flats from various phone boxes and putting the phone down abruptly when they mentioned the Kaltmiete. *I found a flat in the end. When my stepmum tells me stories about paying off her mortgage of two and six a week by selling potatoes from door to door in a broken pram, this is how you guys feel when we year 2000 expats tell you all about our seven-room flats in Prenzlauer Berg for 150 marks a month and it had TWO balconies but, unfortunately, a* Dusche *in the* Küche *and* Ofenheizung. *We know how jealous and mad it makes you. But we just can't stop!*

How I Gentrifiziert Myself Weg

So, when I arrived in Germany, there were still DMs – *Deutschmarks*, as we said (wrongly?) in English.* And Berlin was cheeeeeeeeaop in those days. When the bill came at the end of the evening in posh restaurants in Charlottenburg, me and my impoverished student friends from Britain literally paid it AND TIPPED like we were in a hiphop video, just notes and testosterone and pure joy and triumph everywhere. I rented a three-room apartment on Kantstraße for 500 marks – and loads of German people told me I was being ripped off!

"But it's five minutes away from the U-Bahnhof!" I told my new German friend, Elise.

"Everywhere in Berlin is five minutes away from the U-Bahnhof," Elise replied blithely. Which was true. In those days, everywhere in Berlin was five minutes away from an underground station. Nobody lived in Plänterwald yet.

What's happened? Now, twenty years later, literally the only people who find rents in Berlin cheap are, like, literally from New York and stuff.

"The greatest thing about this city is how cheap it is!" my New York friend, Tina, says. "It's soooooooooooo cheap. I mean, have you seen my place? It is beautiful, isn't it. It's practically a

---

* Wrongly, indeed: "Deutsche Mark" ist the correct plural of "Deutsche Mark". — German editor

palace. I basically live in Versailles. And there's an U-Bahn station just, like, three minutes away! And I'm not even paying 2000 euros a month! Can you believe it?"

It's easy to blame Tina – it's easy to blame myself, even – for the rising rents. Isn't it? And I WAS a dickhead in 2000. It was ignorant and *unsolidarisch* of me to not find out how much I should be paying for a flat and refuse to pay a penny more. It's unsolidarisch of people to go on and on and ON and ON and ON and on about how cheap they find their flats in Berlin – when literally just ten years ago, working-class people could live in the centre of town (I don't mean the centre of town, as in Mitte, the swanky borough of Mitte, I mean the centre of town as in inside the Ring, the S-Bahn line that circles Berlin), and now there are ordinary middle-class people struggling to find small affordable flats near their kids' school. People shouldn't be flippant, and they shouldn't be too grateful. Still, though. The housing crisis in Berlin has been exacerbated by expats' generosity, flippancy, and over-the-top gratitude – it hasn't been caused by it. The problem was the *Senat* selling off all the social housing. They need to sort their fucking lives out.

There was a rental cap a couple of years back, which got overturned by the court of appeals. Everyone is constantly assuring me that landlords aren't evil but they just can't survive without charging people exorbitant rents. Well, if that's true, that's really sad isn't it, and a bit of a shame, because people have to live somewhere and we'll just have to have the state provide us with social housing. Vienna should be our role-model. And "500 Mark Dreizimmerwohnungen für alle – not just people with time travel abilities" should be our slogan.

* * *

Kartoffel: *Yummy delicious wonderful potatoes. I love potatoes. Mashed potatoes are* Kartoffelbrei. *Boiled potatoes are* Salzkartoffeln, *yummy yummy.* Bratkartoffeln *can be roast potatoes or fried potatoes.* Kartoffelpuffer *are these weird very thin hash brown thingies.* Bauernfrühstuck *is just the yummiest thing you will ever eat in your life, i.e.* Bratkartoffeln *with tiny chunks of bacon hidden inside, deliciously.*

Kartoffel *is also a mocking term – I wouldn't even call it an insult to be honest – for white German people. They're surprisingly sensitive about it, actually. Like, I can think of worst things to be called? Kartoffeln are really delish, you guys.*

Krautspeak

Even after all my years in Germany, my family can't really believe I speak German. It's weird to them. When I go home, at some point in the night, they put World War II documentaries on, and I stand next to the telly, so I can't see the subtitles, and say what the old Nazis are saying in English, and everyone compares what I say with what the Nazis are saying and murmurs approvingly.

"It's like you know every word," my mum says. "Almost."

"Your krautspeak's really good," my aunt says.

"You're just so fluent," my mum says. "It's amazing really. Why don't you phone the German government up and tell them how good your German is? Maybe they could get you a job as a civil servant or something. Or what about the German BBC? Or the German FA? I'm sure they could find a position for you."

I don't have the heart to tell her that every German under the age of 35 speaks far better English than I do German. I just nod vaguely.

"Would you say krautspeak is a harder language to learn than English?" my auntie says.

My mum nods at Ryan surreptiously and hisses at my aunt: "Stop calling German krautspeak. You'll hurt his feelings. It's hate speech."

Ryan looks at her blankly. He is just waiting patiently for it to be his turn to stand next to the TV translating the old Nazis.

"Actually, I don't think Ryan even knows the Germans are called krauts. Do you?" I ask him.

"Yeah," he says vaguely. "You say it all the time. I thought it came from *crowd*, though. Nana, let me translate the Nazis for you!"

Ryan does it with his eyes closed, for extra impressiveness, and my parents clap him. Well my aunt claps and my mum cheers.

My aunt says: "He's even better than you, Cinty."

"So, what do the krauts call us, Ryan?"

Ryan looks at me worriedly.

"In Germany, the bad word for Germans is *Kartoffel*," he says, tactfully. My parents aren't interested, though.

"Come on, you can tell us," they say. "We won't be offended."

Ryan says quietly: "Island monkeys."

Silence descends. Well, except for the sound of a World War II doku in the background, of course.

"Island monkeys!" My mum says, genuinely offended. "Now that really is hate speech."

"It's not meant in a bad way," I say. "They just think we're backward and ugly."

"Maybe island apes," Ryan says. "Is island apes better?"

"I'm not going to feel guilty about calling them krauts anymore," my aunt says.

"Oh!" Ryan says. "Because of *Sauerkraut*!" He starts

laughing. "You know that is really funny," he says. "British people are so funny, especially when they're insulting Germans!"

And you know what? That is probably one of the most German sentences he has ever said.

* * *

Kirchensteuer: *Another composite noun, yay.* Kirchen – *church* – Steuer – *tax. Put 'em together and what do you get? The very weird medieval-sounding church tax. Well, guess what? It's as medieval as it sounds – people who believe in God have to literally put their money where their mouths are.*

Church Tax: Is This the Weirdest Thing About Life in Germany?

"So, this weird thing happened," says my friend Charlotte, who has literally been living in Germany since, I dunno, SHARKS EVOLVED.

"What?" I say.

"I was looking at my pay slip – you know how I am freelance but I still get a pay slip because erm. I'm kind of not freelance?"

"I know," I say.

"So I was looking at my pay slip and I noticed like all this money was going. Like it was just being like, taken off of me. Like all this extra money. Quite a lot, actually."

"Really?" I say.

"So, I phoned up my tax guy," she says.

"He's stopped ghosting you?" I say.

"Kind of," she says. "But anyways, guess what?"

"What?"

"IT WAS CHURCH TAX!" she wails desperately and I collapse into hysterical laughter.

"Stop it, Jacinta!" she barks at me. "Stop it! Stop it. Stop it now. Stop it. Shut up. That's my money. That's money I could've been spending on my kid. Stop it. Stop it. Jacinta. Stop it. This is why people hate you so much, you know that?"

I try to stop laughing as tears of pure schadenfreude literally cascade down my face and then I whisper: "Charlotte, why the fuck did you tell the Finanzamt you were Christian, you fucking idiot? You didn't even know what Ascension Day was until I told you!"

"I didn't, they just decided I was for some reason."

"How much money was it?" I whisper.

She whispers back: "Like over the years? Thousands. Thousands."

I start laughing again. "You thought Jonah the whale guy was the same person as Noah the ark guy!"

"I did not," she snaps. "I thought they were like brothers or something? They both, like, hang out in water a lot?"

"You called Noah's ark a boat!" I cry.

"Well, it is a boat, isn't it," she says sulkily. "What is it, if it's not a boat? It's not a fucking aeroplane, is it!"

"Why'd the Finanzamt decide you were Christian? What's that about?"

"I have no idea," she says. "Fucking bastards. First the priests rape all these little boys, and then the bastards start robbing impoverished single mothers ..."

"You're not exactly penniless if your church tax is in the thousands," I say, reasonably. "What is it? Nine per cent or something?"

"What are they spending all their fucking church tax on anyway," she says crossly. "Every time I'm on holiday and I go in a fucking cathedral it's costing me a euro to light a fucking candle!"

I stop laughing long enough to feel guilty for having laughed at my friend's situation so badly. She is right, this is why people hate me so much. I breathe in empathy and kindness and stuff like that. And then I say, seriously: "I think, to be fair, the money does go to good causes. Like I know loads of white Germans who don't leave the church because they think they owe all the good causes that money. Like you know that *Frauenhaus* I was in? That was a Caritas *Frauenhaus*. It's not all stained-glass windows and cushions and that."

"I just can't believe it! You know who I think grassed me up? When I first arrived in the country, and I went to go and get *angemeldet*, the lady in the *Meldeamt* was all like are you Christian? I thought she was, like, making small talk. And I said to her, no I have never been christened but I went to a Catholic high school. That fucking bitch. I thought she was making conversation. I thought she was being friendly for the sake of it!"

"Let this be a lesson to you Charlotte. These People. Are. NEVER. Friendly. For the sake of it!"

So, as you guys know, I am a SJW extraordinaire and as such am fully signed up to the belief that you can't be racist towards white people (I do try my hardest though). BUT I gotta say: church tax is one example of non-white privilege I think. Apparently there are non-Christian communities/parishes in Germany that can claim something like church tax, e.g. Jewish *Kultussteuer*, but generally speaking it seems to me like it is mainly a Christian thing, and it seems to me like it's very, very unusual for a PoC-expat (seems like an oxymoron, lol) to get sneakily hit with the dreaded church tax, just because they went to Brownies for three years in the 1980s. But I have loads of white friends who have suffered in this way, and once I stop laughing at them, I think it's terrible. (By the way, German Beamtes haven't realised that there are non-white Christians yet).

My personal opinion is that church tax or *Kirchensteuer* is a fucking travesty and if you're going to do it, at least be upfront about it – and believe people when they say they aren't officially Christian. And, whilst it is nice that Christians basically seem to have accepted that nobody believes in God anymore, and so have decided to spend their time and energy doing nice Christian deeds involving soup kitchens and intercultural single mum breakfast clubs and setting up schools and that, it's a bit weird that Germans are so judgy about Muslim countries when the two main Christian churches are SO involved in daily German life? And I also find it super-weird that Germans spend so much time of every day wittering on about what a *Sozialparadies* Germany is, a country where it is basically, unlike the US or the UK, IMPOSSIBLE to become homeless, when basically if every single Christian in the country woke up and admitted to themselves that God probably doesn't exist, this country would be totally fucked. I think there should be state-run, ATHEIST women's refuges, homeless shelters and soup kitchens – maybe a few Christian and Muslim ones AS DECORATION – but the basic infrastructure should be provided by the state and atheist AF. Also, I'd ban religious schools and make *Religionsunterricht* neutral. But this is all just my personal opinion, and to be honest, I don't really care that much.

However, whatever you do: IF YOU ARRIVE IN GERMANY DO NOT MAKE SMALL TALK WITH THE MELDEAMT LADY! Do not tell her about singing Sing Hosanna in assembly or the time you had hallucinatory sex with Jesus on magic mushrooms. Tell her your high school was basically North Korea mixed with Sweden, tell her every wedding you've ever been to has taken place in a school gym, tell her you're a pagan, TELL HER NOTHING. You think she is a sweet German Beamtin trying to make small talk but actually she wants to rob you blind.

* * *

Kita: *In Berlin, a nursery school is always called a* Kita *– short for* Kindertagesstätte. *If you hear someone saying* Kindergarten, *that's just like when Brits call the pharmacist a chemist. But, annoyingly, this isn't true for the whole of Germany. In Munich, for example, you go to* Kita *until you're three, and to* Kindergarten *from three until six. Sometimes I seriously don't know how anyone is ever meant to learn this language!*

Ignorance Is Bliss

Am listening to a podcast when my littlest son asks me: "What's ignorant?"

"Oh," I say. "If you don't know something, that means you're ignorant."

"Like me with all the words," he says sadly.

"Yeah," I agree.

"There are so many words I don't know," he says.

"It's okay," I say.

"I am igerwent," he says.

"You used that perfectly," I say.

"I am so igerwent, I don't know the dwiffwence between a Kita and a Kindergarten."

It's funny isn't it. Here in Germany, people are always complaining about Denglisch words – but nobody in the UK minds *Kindergarten*. Although it really isn't as simple as saying *Kinder-*

garten is used in the English language as a German word for nursery. It's really not that simple. In Britain, posh people use it for the little kids' part of a posh private school. In the States, it's the reception class at primary schools. And in Australia, it really is used for nursery school – and they shorten it, adorably, to *kindie*.

When I first started teaching English at German *Kindergartens**, the word *Kita* was new and my *Sachbearbeiter* at the Jobcenter – or my case worker at the dole office – wouldn't let me use the word *Kita*. "Such a beautiful young girl shouldn't have such an ugly West word in her mouth!" he'd say lovingly.

He really loved me that guy. Once I heard him talking about me on the phone and he made me sound like one step up from a dead rat. "Yes," he said, "she has a degree – but it's in German, and she can't speak German. So it's basically worthless! And her German is really bad – there are Turkish grandmas who speak better than her. She is a single mother, basically unqualified, no German skills, nothing going for her – but she needs our help. If anybody needs our help, it's this girl!" I felt like some kind of impoverished street urchin.

Nowadays, everyone mainly says *Kita*, but every now and then *kindergarten*. I'd compare it to how often my mum said cinema versus how often she said pictures. Or swimming pool and baths!

Even though kindergarten doesn't actually mean nursery school in British English, none of my British rellies ever asked me or Ryan or Leo what we actually mean when we say *Kita* or *Kindergarten*. My mum did ask me once, though, what *Kita* actually meant.

"What does *Kita* actually mean?" She asked.

"It's an abbreviation," I said.

---

* The correct plural is "Kindergärten". — German editor.

"Is it short for keetamine?" she asked. I was surprised that she had heard of it, and even more surprised that she thought Berliners, or Germans, would name their daycare institutions after the drug.

"No," I said.

"Must be short for something," she said.

"It's short for *Kindertagesstätte,*" I said.

"I don't know what that means," she answered. "I don't speak German."

Since my mum died, I'd give anything to have one of these bewildering conversations with her again, but at the time, I was quite perplexed by it all, to be honest.

Now I turn the podcast on my phone off, walk out of the kitchen, pick my son up and throw him on his bed.

"You're not ignorant!" I say. "You're just learning!"

"I don't learn any letters in Kita," he whispers, as if his Erzieherin could hear him all the way over here. "I learn all my letters from you or YouTube."

"I know," I say. The truth is, I can be a bit of a hot-houser sometimes. It comes naturally to me.

* * *

Koch: *In English, a cook is someone who cooks for fun, or as a "job." My aunt who works at a school, heating up dinners for school dinners, and my cousin who works at an old people's home, they are cooks. A chef is a qualified cook – someone with professional training. Nigella Lawson, for example, a famous TV chef, is always emphasising the fact that, actually, she isn't a chef at all – but a cook.*

There's no such distinction in German. If you're a Koch *– or a* Köchin *– it's assumed you'll have some form of qualifications. And if you're just someone who loves cooking, you can call yourself a* Hobbykoch.

It all gets a bit confusing because Chef *means boss in German. Although most Germans will probably recognise the word boss, most English speakers don't know that the German word for boss is* Chef. *Also, there is no word for bossy in the German language – something that really annoyed me when reading "The Corrections" by Jonathan Franzen. My theory is that Germans are SO bossy, they don't need a word. It's like the opposite of Eskimos and snow – Germans are so bossy, that's just their default personality type.*

The Worst Cooks in Europe: A Rap Battle

Germans are always slagging off the British for being bad at cooking – but we know it's just to distract attention away from their own culinary disasters.

The first time I ever got invited to a German's for dinner, they served me pasta with a tomatoey-tuna sauce. It was fine. It was perfectly fine. It was absolutely okay. It was almost nice. I mean, it was quite nice. It was just nothing special.

"I bet you've never tasted anything like this before, have you, Jacinta?" Lutz said to me, grinning provocatively.

"What?" I said.

"I bet you've never had anything like this cooked for you before, have you?" he grinned.

"Erm," I said.

"We all know about the British and cooking! The British can't cook, the British don't cook!" He laughed cheerfully at his hilarious comment.

"We have tuna," I said to him. "We have tuna in Britain. We have tuna and pasta. That's a thing we eat."

The Germans and the British are probably the worst cooks in Europe, huh, and we both try to distract attention away from our own shit culinary skills by pointing out the other's weakness. I have to admit to finding it annoying, a little bit. I am a bit of a foodie – actually maybe I am a bit of a fattie – and a huge part of my homesickness is inspired by my hunger pains. I miss English food. I wake up every Saturday craving a fry-up, and every Sunday craving a roast chicken with Yorkshire puddings and mash. I LOVE English food. There, I said it. I love it all. I love having chips with everything – big, gorgeous, golden, perfect chips, which, when made to perfection, which at the fish & chip shop my cousin works at they almost always are – manage to be slightly soggy and perfectly fluffy at the same time (HOW?), I love having lasagne and chips, I love fish and chips, I love sausage and chips, I love battered sausages and I love chipolatas. I love it all. I also love pies and I love the way the Asian community just totally culturally appropriates pies and you can get a chicken tikka pie as well as a steak and kidney pie if you so wish. I love peri-peri chicken. I love ham, egg and chips. I love a Sunday roast, I love bubble and squeak, I love toad-in-the-hole, I love shepherd's pie, I love it all. I LOVE IT.

Germans think British people can't cook for the following reasons:

1. We are a bit shit at cooking, compared to everywhere-else-in-Europe, except for Germany, to be fair.
2. London is so expensive, and Germans just meander around these awful tourist places and pay 50 quid for a lump of reheated fried chicken and chips that you can't actually swallow. This is unfair, I feel. London is the only city in the world where the tourist crap gets seen as representing the national cuisine.
3. Germans have these weird, slightly racist ideas in their heads about proper cuisine and traditional cuisine and En-

glish cuisine, and are also super-pussyish re spicy food. So they're not prepared to eat any Indian food when they visit Britain, they don't even try the culturally appropriative pies, and then they complain about how shit the food is. It's ridiculous.

4. Brits are poorer than Germans, huh? On average. There are more poor people, cooking badly, and eating crap. Because of poverty, it's hard to eat well when you don't have enough money. And a lot of those poor people take on German exchange students in Bournemouth to make a bit of extra money. And as we all know, Germans are seriously fucking traumatised by their Bournemouth school exchanges.
5. Germans really care about what food looks like, and British people like to pile it all up into one glorious, gorgeous, stodgy, delightful mess.
6. Germans worry really far too much about fried food, especially since they literally all live off a diet which is 90 per cent salami, nine per cent Bockwurst and one per cent three-day-old wilted cucumber. You might as well fry a bit of bread if you're gonna load up on pork like that anyway.

What I will say, though, is that British people cook more than Germans realise, and slightly more exuberantly. British men cook more than German men. Ethnic minorities mix the foods up more – mix up traditional British cuisine with their own culture's dishes and the people who do cook actually enjoy cooking more (this isn't the most scientific thing I ever said). Also people invite each other over for dinner more – it IS galling being constantly told how shit you are at cooking by people who you've known for seven years and you've never even gotten a fucking sandwich out of the stingy bastards, and yes, if you know me in real life and feel *angesprochen* right now, this is undoubtedly a dig at you.

ALSO POSH BRITISH PEOPLE COOK WELL AND HEALTHY AND POSH, as posh people should, *Bio* and that. What is the point of being posh if you're not going to eat truffles and quails' eggs and stuff and have organic bread? Like I have some posh German friends, architects and stuff, who let their kids have Nutellabrot for tea and the bread they use is Sammy's Sandwich Toast and not even the Sammy stuff, but the supermarket own brand. I think it's amazing that even posh Germans will feed their kids crap. I really don't think they should judge us that much, to be honest.

* * *

Kopftuch: Kopf *means head and* Tuch *means scarf/cloth covering so put them together and what have you got? That's right: the headscarf. Germans are plain weird about the headscarf. Like, think of the most racist English speaker you know, with the ugliest, most paranoid thoughts about why some women might want to, for religious or maybe even, let's be honest, cultural reasons, cover up the hair on their heads, times the hate-filled paranoia by a thousand and you'll be somewhere close to the mainstream white German opinion on headscarves.*

German Feminists and the Headscarf: The Dictionary Definition of Very Fucking Weird

"So I made this new feminist friend, huh," my friend Lola tells me. "She is my age and she is so cool!"

Lola is 26 and like all people who are under thirty, she thinks it matters what age you are. Like, really matters. Like, it has something to do with you, really, like getting old is this terrible choice people make and they should just say no, like she will, and remain 29 forever. Seriously, I don't want to be a grumpy old woman about this, but I was no cooler ten years ago than I am now. I was pretty fucking uncool ten years ago, to be honest. I still, ten years ago, actually preferred pop music to proper music and found nightclubs a bit stressful. But somehow, because you get older, because time goes forward, literally goes forward, young people act like they're being really generous for hanging out with you even though there's the number 80 on your birth certificate. Someone should tell them that age ain't nothing but a number! It's a bit annoying to be honest.

"Oh, that's nice," I say. "You should have more feminist friends. They're good for you."

"She is so nice," Lola says, happily. "Totally nice and completely feminist. Rape, abortion you name it. Oh!"

Lola suddenly looks kind of crestfallen.

"There's just one thing she's weird about."

"Headscarf?" I say, nodding lots. I've been in Germany one million years now. I am ancient after all. I know what kind of things German feminists are weird about.

"Headscarf," she says, nodding lots.

"Does she think it's okay, the teacher ban?"

Lola looks kind of embarrassed.

"I think if she had her way, they'd ban everyone from wearing it – even women who work in, like, headscarf shops and stuff."

German feminists and the headscarf. It's weird, man. I actually think that a German feminist can be anti-headscarf and not actually be a total Islamophobe. If anyone from the UK or the US felt the same way, you know, I'd strike them off my Christmas list. But if you struck every anti-headscarf German feminist off your Christmas card list (which doesn't exist because you live in Germany and everyone here is too grown-up and sensible to send Christmas cards) you wouldn't have many German feminist friends left. Also, the thing is, I really think the headscarf is seen differently in their heads than it is in ours.

The thing you have to understand is that their feelings about the headscarf are very clear. They are tangible – and they see the headscarf as tangible too. Very absolute. They see this headscarf – the wish some women have to not show their hair in public – as only sexist. ONLY sexist. Just oppression. It's basic as fuck of them, but that is what they see. They see women in hijab as if they're walking around with a sign on their foreheads saying "OPPRESSION IS GOOD". This is what the headscarf is for German feminists. Like it is purely, 100 per cent only a sexist symbol. This is why you will find, after you have lived here a while, that you will have German feminist friends who will be totally, completely and absolutely normal on every other topic, but who want to ban the headscarf or, at the very least, find the ban for teachers okay. And you know what else? Not all of them will be grannies like me. Some of them will be pretty fucking young.

I can see why people think the headscarf is sexist, by the way. It's only women who cover their hair, not men, so therefore, they say, the headscarf is fundamentally sexist. I don't completely understand why other things which only women wear and not men – skirts, high heels, foundation – shouldn't be banned too but there you go. Well, I do understand, really. High heels, which are actually really fucking dangerous for your feet, are as much of a symbol of oppression as the headscarf (if a headscarf is oppressive). However, they are not seen as foreign. They're not seen as imported oppression. This is why you have to search pretty fucking high and wide before you find a German feminist who wants to ban high heels.

The thing is this, though. Women should be free to choose what they want to wear. Women in Iran and Saudi Arabia should be free to show their hair in public – and women in the West should be free to cover up. It's actually pretty sexist that men are allowed to go swimming with their nipples showing. But this sexism wouldn't make it okay for people to force women to reveal their nipples, too. That's not freedom, that's not equality.

One thing I have never understood about the anti-headscarf stance is the whole religious symbol stuff. Of course, the headscarf is a symbol, and it's a symbol connected to a religion, but it's not a religious symbol in the way a cross is. There are lots of Muslim women who don't wear a hijab, just like there are lots of non-Muslim women who wear headscarves – the Queen and nuns, for example (the latter of which strangely ARE allowed to teach in German schools. Go figure). The other thing I don't understand is why it's okay for kids to see women in headscarves cleaning the school after the bell rings for the end of the day – but not okay for them to be taught by them? There's never actually been this ban of the headscarf in educational settings people think there has. What there has been though, is the German state doubling down on women it thinks are so oppressed that the only way to end this oppression is to ban them from teaching.

When I came to Germany, aged twenty, I got used to a lot of things quickly. I stopped sending Christmas cards the second Christmas I spent out here – look, it's a stupid tradition okay? But it's taken me nearly twenty years to understand the German feminist position on the headscarf – and I am not sure if understand is the right word, really. But maybe it's time for German feminists to do a bit of thinking too?

* * *

Kur: Kur *means, I mean, you probably guessed it – cure. But* eine Kur *normally means a kind of basic wellness retreat/rehab holiday – but not the kind that millionaire junkies/supermodels go on. It's like rehab for normal, ordinary people, with normal ordinary health problems which they can "cure" or recover from, I guess – at the* Kur. *It's paid for by your* Krankenkasse *– health insurance provider. The most famous ones in my circle of friends are the* Mutter-Kind-Kurs* *– mother and child retreats. White Germans are always lecturing you about how many* Kurs *you're entitled to how often, posh expats say you have to persuade your doctor and your insurance company into it – most Ausländer steer clear and just pay to go to* Tropical Islands *instead.*

Horrific, Traumatic Kur Experience

My British Asian friend, Anni, fought for like three years to get her Kur bewilligt – given the green light, basically. And on her first night at the Kurhotel, she rings me up to complain.

"It's literally like prison here," she says. "You should see the beds. They're like wooden beds like fucking prison or something."

"Oh," I say.

"They should reappropriate these places next *Flüchtlingskrise,*" she says darkly. "Nobody is racist enough to begrudge the refugees this kind of accommodation. And the food! It's like hospital food! Like grey bread and margarine and turkey ham."

"Oh," I say.

"And one wilted cucumber," she says.

"Oh," I say.

"I want to die," she says. "I hate it here."

---

* "Kuren" is the correct plural. — German editor

"You'll probably do, like, physiotherapy tomorrow," I say encouragingly.

"The rooms are cold," she says. "I'm cold. My kids are cold. I hate it here. What am I doing with my life? I'm going to need a fucking Kur," she spits emphatically, "to recover from this fucking Kur."

"Are the other mums nice though?" I ask weakly.

"Oh God, that's the worst thing," she says. "All the other mums are German!" she sighs. "Probably it's only German mums who are masochistic enough to put up with this shit. I fought so hard to get my Krankenkasse to pay for this! I should've just spent that time doing overtime, saved the extra money, and taken us on an all-inclusive trip to Majorca."

"Think about the breakfast buffets they have at places like that," I say, somewhat unhelpfully.

"Oh fuck off, Jacinta," she says and hangs up on me and I don't hear from her for another three months, which is, when you think about it, fair enough, probably.

Chapter Twelve:

L is for …

Latzhose: Latzhose *are dungarees, and* Hosenträger *are braces (or, as Americans call them, suspenders.) My teen used to call* Latzhose *"Latztrousers" and* Hosenträger *"trousers-carriers", but he's grown out of it now.*

Sauna-Hose

When my teenager Ryan was a little boy, we didn't have much money, so he always wore hand-me-downs. Sadly for him, a lot of these hand-me-downs were dungarees, which he didn't like. He wanted to wear cool trousers – *coole Hose* – i.e normal ones, and not *Sauna-Hose,* which for some reason, and I had no idea why, was what he called dungarees. Every morning, I fought with him like mad to get him into his dungarees. Looking back, I wish I had just gone shoplifting, to be honest, or to a second-hand clothing store, got him a load of normal trousers and been done with it. But guess what? My kids get their stubbornness from me, and I didn't do this and we fought every morning.

And then one morning we were late for Kita because we had been fighting so much.

"I'm sorry we're late," I said. "It took me ages to get him into his dungarees."

I knew the word for dungarees – *Latzhose*.

And then I asked the nursery school teacher.

"Do you know why he thinks people wear dungarees in the sauna?"

She looked at me blankly.

"*Sauna-Hose*," I explained. "He always wants to wear *coole Hose*, and not *Sauna-Hose*. I always thought German saunas were naked."

She then laughed at me non-stop for approximately 45 minutes – I have seldom seen a German so happy – and explained that he was, in fact, calling *Latzhose "so 'ne Hose"* short for *"so eine Hose"* in other words, trousers like that.

Now he's a teenager and cooler than ever. He'll only wear Levis and T-shirts from Gucci or Armani (luckily for me, they can be fake though. He goes to school in Neukölln, not Wilmersdorf). But we don't fight about it anymore. I've realised there's no point trying to save money if your kid's coolness is at stake.

Chapter Thirteen: M is for ...

Migrationshintergrundler: *Germans don't see race, which is kind of fucked-up, and kind of understandable, to be honest. The understandable bit is that they think if they start seeing race, they might become Nazis again. The fucked-up bit is that they do see race really, they just never admit they do.*

It's only very recently that German people started using the word white. When I arrived here, in the year 2000, you were either German, or not German. And people stayed Turkish – or Ausländer *– forever. I remember an article in* Tip *or* Zitty, *in the early 2000s, blithely asserting that an area where a lot of "Ausländer" lived was a problem area – a* Problemviertel. *Okay, so first up, maybe people who aren't German shouldn't be automatically equated with problems, huh – but the really galling thing is, probably most of the "Ausländer" they were referring to were born and bred in Germany!*

So, a new word was needed. First of all people said Bürger mit Migrationshintergrund *– Citizens with a background of immigration. This is admittedly a bit of a mouthful, so before too long, it got shortened to* Migrationshintergrundler.

Of course, the thing is, if people want to be racist, they can just say Migrationshintergrundler *and mean* Ausländer. *To be honest, they can say* Migrationshintergrundler *and mean* Kanake *(a pretty offensive word for brown people).*

This is as good a place as any to mention the great Ausländer/ex-

pat divide. In recent years Germans have started saying, also when speaking German, expat. They use it to mean posh Ausländer – people with degrees, and white skin and lots of privilege. The weird thing is, though, that a lot of Syrians who arrived in 2015 also call themselves expats, and nobody can correct them (it would be a bit rude to go, actually, you're not expats, sorry) and so the whole expat/Ausländer distinction is dying out a bit.

The Syrians who arrived in 2015 are really refugees. Some Germans even use the word refugees when speaking German. The proper words are Flüchtlinge or Geflüchtete, Geflüchtete sounds a bit nicer. You must never say Asylanten and Asylbewerber is just for official usage.

What's really missing in the German language is a name for people who don't look German. People say PoC, the American word, when speaking German. I'll admit it feels funny doing so when the people we are referring to – Turks and Arabs – are often so pale that they look white. After I'd been living in Germany for a few years, and I started calling white British people "British" or "English", my friends from school thought I'd turned totally racist – but they also find it weird that I don't think Turkish people are white anymore.

Race is a minefield in Germany. One of the biggest problems when talking about race or racism is that there isn't even a word for race. The German word Rasse really is more Nazi and more genetic and more weird than race. You can't talk about someone's Rasse without turning them into a dog at best, or measuring their skull's circumference at worst. What a lot of people do is just use the English word race when speaking German. This is what I do, mainly. Sometimes people exchange race for Hautfarbe, like for example when Reni Eddo-Lodge published "Why I'm No Longer Talking to White People About Race", in Germany, they translated "Warum ich nicht länger mit Weißen über Hautfarbe spreche". All of these solutions are unsatisfactory – had I been the publishers, I would have given the book a completely different title, I think.

People will often try telling you, if you find anything racist, that you just "don't understand" German history. It's total crap, of course. The Holocaust having happened is no excuse for the discrimination of Germans of Turkish and Arabic origin experience in everyday life. It can sometimes seem like there are white Germans (liberals as well, I'm not even getting into the AfD people – or the Querdenkers) out there who think the worst thing about the Shoah is that it has made Germans not racist enough towards their immigrant communities.

One of the most controversial opinions I have is that Germany is a far less racist country (and it's still racist as fuck) than the country I arrived in twenty years ago. You don't hear middle-class people claiming Turkish people steal, or Arabic people smell, anymore. It's weirdly more Nazi but less racist, on the whole. Still, racism in Germany is a huge problem – and not having a word to describe those Migrationshintergrundler *who get treated like* Migrationshintergrundler *no matter how good their spoken German might be – is part of the problem.*

Germany: If You Don't See Race, You Can't See Racism

Here's a list of things, possibly incomplete, that white Germans have told me are not racist:

1. Sending a Sikh guy who wears a turban an SMS asking him if he will give you a lift home on his magic carpet.
2. Not wanting to give a German-Turkish girl who wears a headscarf an *Ausbildung* at your company.
3. Thinking someone's name sounds silly and telling them so.
4. Banning German-Turkish and/or German-Arab schoolkids

– or even nursery-schoolkids! – from communicating in their mother tongues in the playground.

5. Not wanting to give a German-Arab boy a job at your company, because of course you'd rather employ a *German*-German, it's just easier.
6. Teachers thinking German-Arab and/or German-Turkish kids shouldn't go to grammar schools because their parents are probably stupid.
7. Bus drivers asking only black guys to show their tickets, because, well, they perhaps don't have one.

It's tempting to pretend that racism is an American problem, to look at the pictures of George Floyd's face, to watch the videos of his death, and to feel outraged as if the problems of racism are so exotic ...

I don't want to sound like I am equating the black American struggle with the experiences of black people in Europe. The way African Americans have suffered is unique – and uniquely terrible. But it's not okay for white Germans to feel outraged by George Floyd's death as if the problems of racism are exotic to us here. It's tempting, perhaps, to pretend that racism is an American problem – we do it in Britain too, by the way. I never learned a word about colonialism in high school. The only thing I learned about slavery was that the British, unlike the Americans, gave it up voluntarily. But I live in Germany and so I am talking about the country I live in. We have our own racism problems in this country, and the biggest is that nobody is prepared to admit that racism exists.

In a weird way, a fucked-up way, the most racist, Trumpy small town in the States could be less racist than some perfect Prenzlauer Berg bubble, one of those German dinner parties full of white people (I think Alice Schwarzer would call them *fortschrittliche Kreise*) who have never experienced racism, don't have any non-white friends, and spend the evening arguing earnestly about integration, and why some integrate so well and some don't and that's so wrong – without giving a thought about the fact it could be a two-way street. Or why Islamophobia is not, officially, racism. Because white Germans say they don't see race, when the truth is: they don't see racism.

White people in Germany should spend less time worrying about whether things are officially racist or not. It's just a word, man. What's going to happen to Germany if we suddenly thought something was racist and it completely wasn't racist? Literally nothing! Imagine if I said muesli was racist. What would happen? Nothing. I'd just be wrong, that's all. There's always gonna be crazy people who think weird things, what about all those people who think *Just One Day* is a good book? It's okay, the world can cope with a few wrong opinions. Racism isn't this weird topic. It's a part of life, and sometimes people will say things are racist that you don't think are racist, and so what? Chill out, man. If they're wrong, they're wrong. It's okay. White Germans need to spend a bit less time Germansplaining about where racism starts and *Diskriminierung* begins and a bit more time listening to brown and black people talking about the ways in which life in this country is hard and uncomfortable.

Why do white Germans need to be right about racism all the time? Why don't they just shut up and *listen*? What harm would come from them sometimes worrying about whether they are being racist or not, instead of having this knee-jerk reaction, nothing to see here, move along swiftly, that isn't technically racism so we must never think about it ever?

To be honest, as someone who is half-white, I worry about whether I am being racist or not a lot. I think this entire post might be racist – I suspect it might be. I think it might be racist for me to even compare German and American racism. It might venture slightly into downplaying territory, downplaying the very specific struggles that young black and brown men face.

I worry about being racist all the time. And you know what happens? Nothing. Sometimes later on I decide I was racist, sometimes later on I look back and laugh at myself. You don't need to be 100 per cent certain about racism all the time. You can be worried. You can be interested. You can be *curious.*

So, I feel like even though I don't have white privilege, I almost do. I have half-white privilege, I have almost-white privilege, I have non-black privilege. I'm uncertain about race sometimes, uncertain about racism. I think it's okay to worry about whether you're being racist.

I have talked a lot about casual racism in this country, the micro-aggressions, so many of which are worsened by the fact that Germans in general don't care about hurting strangers' feelings, racism + bad manners = 74,0000 micro-aggressions every day of the week. But most importantly, let's never forget that there is a serious problem with racism in the German police. The NSU murders taught us that. And the police in Bavaria and NRW, who are refusing to work in Berlin now that we have an anti-discrimination law, which literally just says discrimination is wrong and you shouldn't do it, know they are racist, too.

German coppers are undoubtedly less violent than the US police – but as well as a very nonchalant attitude towards racial profiling, there have been too many non-whites killed in police custody. Oury Jalloh is the most famous of those, but let's also remember Rooble Warsame, Amad Ahmad, Yaya Jabbi, Achidi John, Laye-Alama Condé and William Tonou-Mbobda. May they rest in peace. I wish I could think of a witty, snappy punchline to end this post on, but to be honest I think that's all I have to say. Rest in peace.

* * *

Mülltrennung: *The Germans, being very sensible people, don't talk about recycling, but* Mülltrennung *– separating your rubbish. They're very good at it, although there are lots of rumours flying about about a colleague's neighbour's cousin's boyfriend who works at the* BSR *and all our different rubbish* – Restmüll *(actual trash),* Biomüll *(compost),* Papier *(paper),* Gelber Punkt *(plastics) and* Glas *(glass, obviously) getting incinerated together. I don't believe these urban legends, but I do believe the stories about us selling our trash to India and stuff.*

We also have a Pfandsystem, *which I do actually think the whole world should copy. We pay a ten or fifteen cent deposit on our bottles or cans, which means everyone recycles them even, or this is the beauty of the system, I guess, especially, drug addicts. When they implemented the system I worried about poor people but I guess we've just got used to it by now. Drinks cost about fifteen cents more than they should, basically. You never see these oceans of coke cans littering the parks in Germany like you do in other countries.*

Trashy Mums at the School Gates

There's a sentence people say about life in Berlin which I've never understood. The people who say this are often a bit posher, a bit whiter, and quite a lot cooler than me. This is what they say: "I love living in Berlin! You feel so free here! You can wear whatever you want! Literally nobody cares!"

Okay, writing it out I notice that it's not one sentence, but four. But still, it's four sentences which I don't, for the fucking life of me, understand.

I know what you're thinking. You're thinking, kinda smugly: Jacinta, you understand the sentiment perfectly – you just disagree, that's all.

NO, GUYS.

I LITERALLY DO NOT UNDERSTAND IT ON A FUNDAMENTAL, ALMOST GRAMMATICAL LEVEL.

What the fuck are they on about?

As far as I am concerned, they might as well be saying Jeeparkootafwaschajabipooditoo. Bingabongleeopgaqina. Scheepeppebi. Tinkyexyplettigorbinor.

What. Are. They. On. About?

You really don't need to be in hijab in Hellersdorf to notice that actually people in Berlin really do care about what other people are wearing. At least they do if you are a parent.

"Why is Baby Leo wearing odd socks?" my German friend Jens asked me.

"Oh, I couldn't find matching ones," I said airily. "And anyway, he is too young to know what matching socks even are, so I thought it didn't matter."

"Hmmmmn," Jens said disapprovingly.

"What, Jens?" I said.

"Well, aren't you worried he will get bullied at Kita for being dressed like a Hartz IV-Prole?"

"Jens!" I replied disbelievingly. "He's like, two years old! I don't think the other kids will care if his socks are matching or not!"

"I don't mean by the other kids," he said. "I mean by the nursery staff."

Jens is so paranoid, I told myself as I went to go and fetch Baby Leo from Kita. But in the changing rooms, a granny who was picking up her grandchild decided to tell me where the nearest soup kitchen was – "You can get clothes there, too!" she said pointedly. "Socks for example."

Have the people who think Berliners don't care what you wear EVER met a German granny? I once, in the middle of summer – it was like nearly 40 degrees out there – had my now-teen, then-toddler in these plasticky sandals with no socks on. Those plasticky sandals that are COMPLETELY COMFORTABLE with no socks on. A German granny came up to me in the street and told me my kid needed to wear socks with his sandals. "There, where you come from, people don't wear socks. They can't afford them. You're in Europe now. You need to dress your kid in a European manner."

Okay, so grannies the world over can be a bit judgy, I hear you saying. But I have been ticked off by people my age so many times – more times than I have had cold Abendbrot, let me tell you. One time I put snow trousers on my son, and it was really rain-trousers time – and my friend said to me: "Do you think it's cold enough for snow trousers?" "Not really," I said. "But we left his rain trousers in Kita, and it's a bit too cold for nothing at all, I thought." I have never forgotten the look of pure icy disapproval on her face.

"Was, bitte, hat die Regenhose in der Kita zu suchen?"

This sentence is almost so disapproving it is impossible to translate. It's almost untranslatable. "How could you have forgotten his rain trousers at nursery school?" mixed with "You filthy whore, go and get yourself sterilised as soon as possible!" comes kinda close.

Just think about all the judgy stories in UK tabloids about schools in Britain warning trashy parents not to do the school run in pyjamas anymore. When I read about this, I assumed that these trashy British parents were not actually rocking up to schools in dressing gowns and jim-jams, but doing that infamous lockdown trick of wearing jogging pants for bed and only basically changing out of them on a weekly basis. But I've since seen photos. WE ARE TALKING PROPER PJS HERE.

There's *Mickey Mouse* pyjamas.

There's *Donald Duck* pyjamas.

There's *Paw Patrol* pyjamas.

There's *Ariel The Little Mermaid* pyjamas.

These parents are another level of trashy. They're not just going to drop off and pick their kids up from school in pyjamas. They're dropping them off and picking them up in the slobbiest, slummiest pyjamas on Earth.

It's not just that I think you couldn't do that over here. It's that I think the trashiest Berlin parents wouldn't even dream of doing so.

I also feel like no Berlin parent has ever sent their kid into school or Kita with odd socks on.

"I've thrown out all of Baby Leo's non-matching socks," I tell my German friend Leonie. "He only has black ones now. Black socks always kind of match, don't they?"

"You're not tough enough for life in this city, Jacinta," Leonie says. "You need to get a thicker skin. You need to learn how to tell people to fuck off. He isn't wearing odd socks because you can't find matching ones! He is wearing odd socks because you care about fashion – and matching socks are so last season."

Chapter Fourteen: N is for …

Nikolaus: *Saint* Nikolaus, *otherwise known as Shit Santa, comes on the 6th December (or is it the 5th December? Am always forgetting) and puts candy in your shoes. Obviously this dude must be the same guy as Santa Claus – there can't be two saints with almost the same name who like gifting kids goodies in their shoes/ stockings right? (The original St. Nick must have had a foot fetish, right?) But is he the same guy as Father Christmas?* Der Weihnachtsmann? *I think so, he looks the same, anyway. Some places in Germany have this creepy fairy called* das Christkind, *who has a weird Jesus baby thing going on, creepy as fuck. I'm so glad I am an atheist whenever I remember that this shit exists. Despite having lived here for one zillion years, I still always forget what day Shit Santa is meant to be coming on. I am a bad German mum.*

Santa Speaks

"Is the guy who brings the shoe candy Santa?" my son Leo asks.

"I don't know," I say. Sometimes I resent Germany for making it obvious that Santa, aka Father Christmas, doesn't exist. Not that Leo seems to have noticed how unrealistic any of this is.

"He came to the Kita," Leo says. "He put candy in all the shoes. The teachers say only clean shoes."

"Yeah, they always say that."

"But there were kids with dirty shoes and he didn't notice. Everyone got shoe candy."

Calling it shoe candy makes it seem kind of gross. Like foot fungus or ear cheese, I find the 6th December kind of annoying. I think it's sweet how proud my dad is of remembering it though. Every year on the 6th December he rings us up and wishes us a happy German Christmas! "Father Christmas came to you on the 6th of December!" he says, proudly. "He comes to Germany nineteen days earlier!"

"I think it's weird," Leo says thoughtfully, "that German people think Santa speaks German and English people think Santa speaks English."

"What?" I say. I read a parenting article recently full of advice about not lying to your kids, but just explaining to them that Santa and Father Christmas and *Nikolaus* and everyone are just these fun magical stories people tell, fun games to keep the magic of Christmas alive and stuff.

"Don't you just think that it's weird?" he asks.

If he's cottoning on anyway, I might as well not lie to him.

"Do you ever think," I say, "that maybe Santa isn't real? But just a magical game people do, at the Kita, to make Christmas seem special? And magic and stuff?"

He laughs.

"Noooooo!" He says scornfully. "Where would they buy the candy from? It had a reindeer on it."

* * *

Nummer: *It's really hard taking down phone numbers in German. I still find it hard after all these years. Some people will do the numbers like this – 030 485 123 –* Null, Drei, Null *– and then instead of listing each number individually for some sadistic reason they go 48, 51, 23. AND as if that wasn't hard enough, because the German for 48 is "eight and forty"* (achtundvierzig), *you're totally fucked. You just literally cannot know what the fuck is going on. AND IF THAT WASN'T HARD ENOUGH, some sadistic bastards will really confuse you by mixing up hundreds in there too.*

The only solution is to say: "Können Sie mir die Nummer einzeln aufsagen, bitte?"

But telephone numbers are not as hard as telling the time!

Piece of Cake

So. Lots of people think that being bad at telling the time is an East German thing, but in fact it's a bit like how most Americans say "eeeeeether" but some do say "eyether" and most Brits say "eyether" but some say "eeeeether" and some people say both: IT'S NOT THAT SIMPLE, ACTUALLY. I have met a lot of West Germans who tell the time normally – and who can't understand what they call the "Eastie" way. And I have met a lot of East Germans who tell the time like sociopaths. But I have also met a lot of West Germans from, like, villages, who swear their granny does it the weird way, and, it has to be said, a lot of East Germans, especially younger ones, who say they can't understand the old ways either.

Oh my God, are you sitting comfortably? Let us begin!

Normal Germans, for want of a better word, tell the time like this:

Viertel nach zehn = quarter past ten

Halb elf = half past ten/half ten (bit weird, but you get used to this after about ten years)

Viertel vor elf = quarter to eleven

Okay so this is what, inexplicably, some Germans think: they think time is a cake.

I know, I know. It doesn't make ANY sense. I know. I KNOW, OKAY? They don't just think that time, an abstract concept, is a cake, they also think that 11 o'clock is a cake. I know. I know. I know. Fuck, man. It's just the weirdest thing you will ever hear in your life, ever.

So if 11 o'clock is a whole cake, then a quarter of eleven, *viertel elf*, is a quarter of the clock on its way round to eleven. I know. I know. But that makes *viertel elf* 10:15.

It goes like this:

Viertel elf: 10:15

Halb elf: 10:30

Dreiviertel elf: 10:45

It's such a shame Agatha Christie wasn't German, She could have written some seriously fucked up murder mysteries based on this kind of misunderstanding.

Chapter Fifteen: O is for ...

Opfer: *The German word for victim and the German word for sacrifice are one and the same (interestingly, and somewhat surprisingly, if you do enough linguistic research, i.e. spend five minutes on Google, you find out that the English and even the Latin words for victim used to mean a human sacrifice too).*

Still, in German the words are the same Du Opfer *means you victim! But* ich opfere mich auf *means I sacrifice myself.*

Weirdly, and, to be honest, slightly disturbingly, Opfer *is a straight up insult in modern German. I mean, to be fair, it's not like the word victim has incredibly positive connotations, right? In English we love victim-blaming – we love accusing people of having a victim-mentality – a lot of people who have suffered from domestic or childhood sexual abuse prefer to call themselves survivors than victims. But the word* Opfer *doesn't just have negative connotations – it's a straight-up insult, used by teens all over the country.*

I've checked with every single white German I know, and none of them thinks that this has anything to do with the Holocaust, but I can't shake the feeling that it must do. The myth inside Germany and abroad is that Germany has confronted the Holocaust and its crimes against humanity more deeply than any country ever known on earth. It takes a few years of living here for you to realise that this is kind of true, but also, at the same time, kind of total bullshit. How could it be true? If it were true, every German alive would kill themselves, surely? The confrontation of the past – Vergangenheitsbewaltigung *– has to be superficial in order for life in Germany to be bearable. So, I can't help feeling that* Opfer *being used as an insult has something to do with a kind of exhaustion at thinking about, and a resentment of having to think about, the Holocaust and the crimes Germany committed.*

But it might just be that American TV shows, when dubbed into German, used Opfer *for loser. It might just be that simple, seriously.*

It's also, I must admit, fun to say out loud: Opfer!*

Opfermentalität

"You're such a victim!" my teenage son says to me.

"Thank you for acknowledging my pain," I reply. "It means a lot to me."

"No, I mean it. Like you're such an *Opfer*!"

"Thanks," I say.

"Mum, I'm insulting you!"

I act shocked. "But how is it an insult to be a victim? It's an insult to be a *Täter*, isn't it?"

My son rolls his eyes. "You're so badly integrated," he says. "You don't even know the most basic insults."

"Hmmm," I say.

"Anyway, victim can be an insult in English too?" he asks, his voice not quite as cocky as it was a few moments ago.

"Not really," I say.

"What about victim mentality?" he asks.

"Oh yeah," I say. "That's an insult alright."

There's a lot of toxic positivity going round at the moment

* FYI: "Opfer" and "Täter" (perpetrator) belong to the group of German words (masculine or neutral, ending on -er) where plural and singular are the same, like e.g. "Berliner". — German editor

– it's our other pandemic. I don't really think Germany is that much worse than Britain or the US in this regard. But the viciousness with which people are sneered at and sniggered at and generally torn to pieces – especially poor people, asking for help or support on the internet – in Facebook parenting groups, for example – can be quite distressing. There's this idea, a kind of inverse of the American dream, that because Germany is so stable and so secure and the German welfare state is SO generous, that anyone who fails to succeed here must be really trying to fail. And a lot of the smug comments about how easy it is to be a single mum, how lucky we are to receive Hartz IV, how great it is that disabled students get a free computer off of the government – come from people who, basically, don't know what the fuck they are talking about.

"I don't have a victim mentality," I tell my son. "I have a victim reality."

"You so have a victim mentality," he answers.

"I think if I didn't have a bit of a victim mentality, being a single mum would be really fucking hard," I say. "You and me, we'd just be fighting all the time. You'd have a chore chart! I'd probably make you wash windows and stuff if I wasn't a bit of a victim."

"Oh yeah," he says. "You're probably right. Mum, you're such a victim ... but in a good way."

Chapter Sixteen: P is for ...

Patriotismus: *Patriotism. The big myth in Germany is that people aren't patriotic in Germany. And maybe this used to be true – or maybe there are slightly fewer Brexitty/Trumpy types over here. But to be honest, ever since the World Cup 2006, there's plenty of flag-flying in Germany. And, you know, I think posh Germans are actually far more patriotic than posh Brits or Americans. There's a kind of bitter paranoia that everyone is laughing at Germany loads more than at other countries, a real defensiveness, and expats/foreigners are constantly being admonished for not being "integrated" or "grateful" enough. In fact, commenting on Germany at all is automatically seen as criticism.*

If We Were Allowed ...

My German friend Katja has come over to see me. Katja is East German, an East Berlinerin, a primary school teacher and a tiny bit boring if I am honest. Like, she's my most boring friend. But our kids are the same age and sometimes a boring German friend can come in kinda handy.

"The Germans aren't allowed to be patriotic," she says sadly. "Because of our history."

"The Holocaust," I say.

"Our complicated history," she says.

I don't mean to be flippant about all the deaths that happened during the Nazi times, but I do feel like shouting at her WAS IT REALLY THAT COMPLICATED? OR DID YOU JUST KILL A LOT OF PEOPLE? Germans are always going on about how direct and honest they are, but they can really pussyfoot around their "complicated history".

"I don't really know what Germans really mean when they say they're not allowed to be patriotic," I say tactfully. "Who isn't allowing you? And what would you like to do differently? Like, you know, I have lived here for thousands of years and when I arrived, it was considered uncool to support Germany in the football. But those days are long-gone, aren't they? So what are you, like, specifically talking about?"

"Well, yes!" she says. "The football! We Germans are not allowed to sing our national anthem unless it's for the football."

"But," I stare at her dumbfounded. Like blankness descends upon me. I have never felt more confused by anything anyone has ever said to me ever, except for when I was coming up on MDMA and my friend Christoph told me he was a private detective. "What are you talking about? Why would anyone sing their national anthem unless it was for the football? What are you literally talking about?" I pause. "Are you talking about the tennis?" I ask.

I've never watched tennis in my life, ever. Maybe they sing the national anthem at the tennis? I know when it rains at Wimbledon they have to sing and stuff. Maybe that is what she is talking about."

"You Brits are always singing your national anthem!"

I stare at her. "Are we?" I whisper. Is she right? Have I been away too long? Wait a minute, she can't be right. I don't even KNOW what the British national anthem even IS! We English sing "God Save the Queen" at the football. It's a shit song, though. But we even had the same boring shitstorm about Wayne Rooney not singing the national anthem as there was in Germany about Özil, though my theory was that Rooney was a secret republican. But I don't know what the British national anthem is or even, a bit shamefully, if we have one. "What is the British national anthem?" I ask her. "Do they sing the British national anthem at the rugby?" Are we Britain for the rugby? I think we might be. Fuck. I really need to google this shit. It's basic general knowledge. I wonder if Britain even has a national anthem ...

I do think Germans exaggerate how unpatriotic they are, you know. Don't get me wrong, there are all these idiots in Britain – or in England, I guess – who are totally embarrassing about the flags and their love for the country. And the flags got bigger after Brexit – and sometimes I think they're getting bigger and bigger every day. And the way the pubs are wallpapered in Union Jacks and St George's every time there's a football tournament, the Olympics, or the Queen has a birthday – God, it's embarrassing. Still. Most educated, non-mad British people – like most educated, non-mad US-Americans, by the way – are slightly ashamed of their country and don't know what their national anthem is. I think most non-mad people are slightly ashamed of their country, aren't they? And I don't want to sound flippant again, but if the price you have to pay for the Holocaust is not being "allowed" to be patriotic, – well, no offence, but it doesn't seem like a very high price to pay to me.

"What about British history?" Katja says. "The Brits are not sorry for colonialism at all! The Germans are the only nation who ever actually say sorry for anything!"

"Well, yes," I say apologetically. "But isn't that actually something you should be a bit ... proud of? I'd love the day to come when the British government and, yeah, even British people, actually tried to repair the damage the British Empire did – or even owned up to it. But I dunno. I kind of feel like setting a good example there is more important than being able to sing the national anthem at non-football events."

I suddenly remember how people used to sing "God Save the Queen" in the cinema. They did it in Australia, too. I really think Katja wouldn't like it if Germans suddenly started doing this. In Britain, whenever you go to the cinema, and in the film they're showing there's a scene from the 40s, the people singing the national anthem, everyone in the cinema laughs. It seems ridiculous now.

"There's a lot of things I am proud of Germany for, actually," Katja says, defiantly.

"Are there?" I ask.

"The bread!" she barks at me. "We have the best bread in the world."

"Oh yeah, the bread," I say.

I guess the bread is good, I don't know, though, because we are officially a *Sammy's Sandwich Toast Haushalt*, and the thing is, I would be ashamed, but they sell so much of the stuff I think some Germans must be secretly buying it too.

"The infrastructure," she says.

"I don't know what infrastructure really means," I admit.

"The trains!" she says.

"The trains?" I ask. "You mean like Deutsche Bahn?"

"No, not Deutsche Bahn," she says crossly. "Of course not Deutsche Bahn. Though it could be good if it wanted to be, the infrastructure is there. But I mean the S-Bahn and the U-Bahn and stuff."

"Right," I say.

"*Kindergeld*," she says. "Nowhere else in the world has Kindergeld."

"Erm," I say. "Britain has Kindergeld. It's called child benefit. Not as much as you get here, but we do have it. And France definitely has it, huh? I think France has Kindergeld."

"All the *Geld* you can get here. *Arbeitslosengeld*. All that Geld. No other country in the world looks after its poor like we do."

"Really?" I say. "I think most places in the Western world have some kind of social welfare system. Or am I wrong?"

"Germany's works so well. It's so fair. It really looks after people."

"Yeah," I say uncertainly. I can think of a few people I know who weren't that well looked after, but I don't say anything.

"The way we treat our disabled kids! It's so great here. A disabled child who lives in Germany has as great a life as an able-bodied child in the US."

"Really?" I ask. I feel kind of sceptical about this, my friend who has a disabled kid seems to have a pretty hard life. But I do also think it's super-hard to have kids in the US because of the lack of maternity leave, nursery schools, social welfare (wait a minute! IS THIS INFRASTRUCTURE?) so I don't say anything.

"*Schulpflicht,*" she says.

"Yeah," I say. I don't really like hanging out with my kids enough to ever complain about it (NO OFFENCE KIDS), but I don't really see why Germans think banning homeschooling, even in non-pandemic times is such a great thing for the country. The kind of people who want to do it are generally just soft hippies, I'd just let them get on with it if it were up to me. And it's not like German schooling is this incredibly high standard.

"Racism," she says.

"You're proud of the racism?" I ask.

"No, Jacinta! I'm proud that there is hardly any racism here!"

"What about the police?" I ask.

"Oh yes, of course," she says, misunderstanding. "The German police are great. Not violent like the American police."

"You think there's hardly any racism here?" I ask.

"Well, look at you. Do you think a foreigner whose English was as good – or as bad, I should say – as your German would have a successful writing career in Britain? I rather doubt it, somehow."

"All my German friends in London are super rich and successful!" I say.

"Yes, and their English is perfect, too," she says.

Auwa, I think.

"Our *Kartoffelsalat* is just so delicious," she says.

Potato salad, I think. She's running out of ideas.

"Our parks are amazing," she says.

"What about Görlitzer Park?" I say. I know Katja hates Görli. She grimaces.

"Our swimming pools are just ... I mean they're fantastic, aren't they?"

To be fair, I also love German swimming pools. The cold public ones are so cheap, they're practically free compared to the UK. The posh hot German baths *(Thermen)* are expensive for us over here, but the same price as the council ones back home – if they haven't been shut down. I don't mind the naked ones if the water is hot enough. If I was German, I guess I would be patriotic about the swimming pools. (I think there should be a single mum family ticket, though.)

"They're really good," I say. "They're much better than the swimming pools in Britain."

"Of course they are!" Katja says airily.

Maybe it's a good thing Katja's not "allowed" to be patriotic, I think to myself. Maybe if she was allowed to be patriotic, her head would get so big it would literally explode.

We sit on my sofa in silence for a few minutes. Then I say: "Telly over here's a load of crap, though."

"Oh, yeah," she says. "German TV is really, really bad."

Even Katja thinks so! I wonder who is boring enough to enjoy it?

* * *

Partys: *So a* Party *is a party where you celebrate stuff, and a political party is called a* Partei. *(Insert your own joke about Boris Johnson and getting mixed up between a* Party *and a* Partei *here) Weirdly, for a kid's birthday party you don't need to specify that a party is happening, the word* Kindergeburtstag *is enough, I've never really understood this. Also, other words for Party:* Fest *or* Feier.

Sometimes parties in Berlin can be a bit confusing. If Germans are inviting you, you can't always tell beforehand if it's going to be ketamine and coke or Kartoffelsalat and sticking post-it notes on your forehead and playing Twenty Questions. Actually, a lot of the time what Germans call a Party *we would call a night out on the town, or going clubbing, or a club night.*

However, if you get invited to an Umtrunk *that means there definitely won't be any ketamine!*

A party animal is a Party-Maus, *and can only be a girl. I feel like a party animal might only drink alcohol whereas a* Party-Maus *likes drugs and techno, too.*

Social Butterflies Do It Best: Social Activities During Global Pandemics Can Be a Bit EXHAUSTING

A fairly good friend sends me a WhatsApp message:

"I miss you loads Jacinta!" she writes. "Hope you and your boys are having a good time in quarantine. Or an okay time, at least? Wanna chat tomorrow? Maybe a Skype call?"

I write back: "I miss you loads too!" I wonder if I'm lying or not. I wonder if we would've actually met up, in non-Corona times, and if I don't miss the idea that I COULD meet up with said fairly good friend more than the actual meeting up itself? It's the freedom to flake out on people last minute that I miss more than the actual live social interaction? Sometimes I think I am in prison, and I say to myself "Jacinta, you're in prison!" and then I remember that I am not in actual prison, and go for a walk, outside, maybe even in a tiny bit of nature, and then I see a poster for a concert that obviously never took place or never will take place and I feel so sad, so fucking sad, so fucking FUCKING sad, not because I am in prison, but because I might as well be, not because I would've gone to that concert – but because I miss the freedom of deciding not to go to that concert more than the actual concert itself.

"Skype call tomorrow?" she writes. "Just tell me when!"

"I'm pretty busy tomorrow, actually," I write back.

She responds: "Good one!"

But the weird thing is: I am not even joking.

The thing is, I'm not sure if I am an introvert or an extrovert. I am someone who other people tend to think is quite loud and extroverted and self-confident, but whenever I do those Cosmo quizzes they usually say I am an introvert. I think I am possibly an introvert trapped in an extrovert's body or, perhaps, vice versa. I like people. I like other people. I even quite like a lot of racists and sexists and people like that. I love my family. I like chatting to grannies in the streets. I don't mind hipsters wearing silly clothes and I never get grumpy, in non-Corona times, about people walking too slowly or standing on the wrong side of the escalator. (I do suspect that I am one of the people that other people get grumpy about, in non-Corona times, for walking too slowly/standing on the wrong side of the escalator.) I literally love everyone in my family, even, or maybe, I mean especially, the alcoholics, and I have often had a lot of fun at a party.

But I'm not a total extrovert, it has to be said. I simply love my own company. I love being drunk alone. I know this is a tragic thing to admit to. When my oldest son is at his dad's and my youngest son is asleep, in non-Corona times I mean, I feel so happy. It feels blissful. I am happiest on Facebook arguing with strangers, drinking red wine, and then reading a bit before bed. Pure bliss.

And you know: I don't find other people HELL – but I do find them a bit exhausting sometimes.

So I kind of thought, as an extroverted introvert, or an introverted extrovert, that I would find these Corona times strangely peaceful, you know? When our semi-lockdown was announced, I expected I'd find it peaceful. I thought there would be lots of lonely evenings spent listening to Helen Reddy and blissing out with a glass of red wine in a non-thrush friendly steaming-hot bubble bath.

CHANCE WOULD BE, AND I CAN'T EXPRESS THIS ENOUGH, A FINE THING. I have so much to do, alongside my home-office, home-education and home-cleaning duties, I am also just constantly inundated with fun social activities I literally can't say no to. My social calendar is as full as it ever was. Actually, what am I talking about? My social calendar is fuller than it has ever been.

I have online book club with a set of nerdy Berlin mums, online yoga class with my friend from high school, online meditation with my friend in Prenzlauer Berg, listening partnerships with other frazzled mums from all over the world, online job coaching sessions specifically to deal with any identity crises arising from the Corona crisis, online job coaching sessions non-specifically dealing with any identity crises which just exist generally speaking in my life in general, online podcast club, where not only do I have to take part in the actual podcast discussion but I also have to prepare by listening to said podcast beforehand, online sacred sister circle AND fun Netflix watch parties. AND these are just the things I've said yes to!

The terrible thing about my social calendar now is you can't pretend your kid is sick to try and get out of anything ... sometimes I get filled with the image of myself if I tried to survive Corona as mentally healthily as possible, constantly gardening on the balcony, baking healthy gluten-free scones in the kitchen, home-educating my kids while home-officing at the same time, Skyping with an overwhelmed mum in Atlanta while also taking part in online podcast discussions in another Fenster ... My mum always used to say when I was little: "A woman's work is never done!" Well, in these harrowing times of Corona, I guess maybe we have to update this saying to: "A woman's fun has only just started!"

I have half an hour to kill before my online book club. I'd better google the plot of the book on Wikipedia. I didn't actually have time to read it, obviously, because I'm just so busy, socially, at the moment.

My son points out the window at a group of kids, who probably don't come from the same family, sitting underneath a slide we can see from our window.

"Playground aputt!" He announces gravely.

"Yeah," I say. "I know."

"Das ist naughty!" He says.

"Yeah, it is a bit," I say.

"DAS IST NAUGHTY!" He calls down at them, and I shut the window, move him away. When this is all over I don't want everyone to call me the Stasi-Tante from Number 11 or anything.

I WhatsApp my fairly good friend back. "I can slot you in for half an hour tomorrow at 15.30?" I write. "See you then!"

"Shall we do some Cindy Crawford?" I ask the baby. "Go get your little chair."

"Cindy Crawford is booooooooooooowing," he says. He pronounces boring exactly as he would had I never moved to Berlin, but just the few miles from Ilford to Dagenham. Boooooooooooooooooooowing – gur.

"You wanna do Tracy Campoli?" I say.

"Das one is booooooooooooowing. Dinosaur, please, Mummy."

I put on Dinostories and go get showered. I even shave my armpits and everything. Online book club, I decide, will only be half as much fun if my pits are hairy.

Chapter Seventeen: Q is for ...

Queen: *So, the German for Queen is* Königin, *but our Queen, Queen Elizabeth, sometimes spelt in German with an s, is called* Queen. *You pronounce it like this:* Kveen. *They like her a lot, and if you slag her off, they tell you off for being unpatriotic or a traitor and stuff. I suspect it's because she is German, it secretly gives them the feeling of ruling over us!*

The Only Time a German Granny Was Nice to Me, EVER

German grannies aren't very nice, huh? They're kinda mean. They're kinda mean and bitchy and judgy and stuff. I mean, you get used to them in the end. But then you go back to Britain and people are literally stopping you in the street to tell you their son Graham got divorced but it's okay, he still sees the kids every Saturday and you're like, fuck, now I remember how nice and friendly grannies can be.

"Eine Schrippe, bitte!" I say to the lady in the bakery.

A *Schrippe* is a cheap white roll – I refuse to buy my kid anything better.

"That's a lovely accent," a granny behind me says.

"Thanks," I say.

"What a lovely accent," she says.

"Yes," I say.

"Let me guess," she says. "Dutch?"

I smile. I have never been mistaken for German, well, only once, but the guy was super drunk, possibly even on drugs. For me, being mistaken for Dutch is as good as it gets.

"English," I say.

She beams at me.

"Well then," she says happily. "Your parents have probably phoned you up to tell you the news already! The little baby is there! AND IT'S A BOY!"

What the fuck is wrong with German people? Why do they love our royal family so much? It's seriously sickening. But the worst part is them expecting you to love them, too. It literally makes me feel ill.

On the one hand, this is the first time a German granny has ever tried to make small talk with me in a bakery ever, and I should reward good behaviour. But on the other hand....

"They have not," I say. "Because they are not fucking idiots."

And with that I sweep out of the shop.

Look, Germany, if you love our royal family so much, you can fucking pay for them, alright?

* * *

Quer: Quer, *not to be confused with* queer *(which is never or almost never an insult in Berlin, but means queer in the positive way it is used in English) means across or diagonal.*

But watch out: never ask a Berliner which part of the building the Quergebäude *is. You'll get a thousand different answers – it seems like literally nobody knows.*

Berlin House Numbers Are Designed to Confuse – You Will Never, Ever, EVER Get Used to Them. My Advice? Don't Even Try!

"We do the house numbers differently in Britain," I explained to a German boyfriend once. I hadn't been long in Berlin, a little bit over a year. I'd only ever seen streets with the numbers going 1 – 150 on one side, and the other way down 151 – 300. Like that.

"Yeah?" he said.

"Yes," I said. I took a deep breath, I was going to need all my German skills to describe this shit.

"What do you call numbers like two, four, six, eight? Even? And how do you describe the numbers one, three, five, seven, nine? Odd? Okay." Another deep breath. "On one roadside – here. The even numbers. Two, four, six, eight. On the other roadside – here." I gesticulated the other side of the road and plonked imaginary houses down next to each other. "Here go the odd numbers. One, three, five, seven. Number one is across from number two. Number three is across from number Four. And so on and so on."

I looked at my German boyfriend.

"I don't know why we do it like that," I added, gravely. Another deep breath.

"The numbers go up the same way. In the same direction. Not opposite ways."

I sighed, exhausted, I had literally used up all my German abilities in that conversation. I was spent.

My German boyfriend looked at me, vaguely interested.

"It's like that everywhere else in Germany," he said.

"NO IT ISN'T!" I yelled, horrified I had so completely linguistically exhausted myself on explaining something that wasn't unique to Britain.

"Yeah," he said. "I don't know why we do it like this in Berlin. It's so confusing. But it's not everywhere in Berlin. Some streets still do it the normal way. Haven't you ever noticed?"

The Berlin house numbering system – and really, using the word system is kinda generous here, to be honest – is the most confusing fucked-up house numbering system ever invented. I mean, I am prepared to be proved wrong on this – maybe the system in Ancient Egypt was even more confusing, but I find it hard to believe. Instead of, like nice, normal people, who want people to be able to find the houses they have to go to, dividing the houses into odd and even numbers, on opposite sides of the roads, they slap them down in chronological number like total sociopaths. And then, and then, and then, AND THEN they go up one way and down the other. It's fine if you're at Number 76 and you need to go to Number 85. Absolutely fine. But what if you need to go to Number 350? You literally have to know how long the road will go on for before you can take a wild stab in the dark as to what side of the road the number will be. It's awful. It's probably one of the hardest things about living in this cold, cold, cold city.

And what about the *Hinterhaus, Quergebäude, Seitenflügel* stuff? The first time my parents came to visit me in my house in Neukölln, I called into the intercom: "WE'RE IN THE BACK-HOUSE!"

"What?" My dad shouted.

"THE BACK-HOUSE! The *Hinterhaus*! The behind-house! THE BACK-HOUSE!"

I ran onto the balcony, and when I saw my parents enter the *Hinterhof*, me and my son jumped up and down for joy. When they finally got upstairs, my stepmum said, disapprovingly: "It's a good thing you were on the balcony to greet us, Cint, we didn't have a clue what you were going on about."

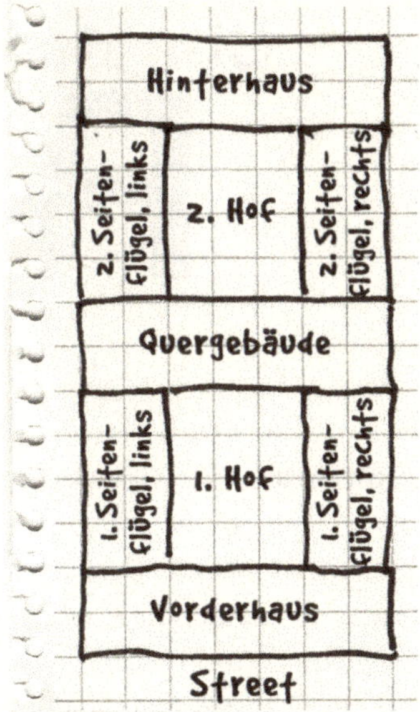

“Well, what’s the English for back-house then?” I asked, sulkily.

“They don’t have a word for it,” my dad said. “Do they? They just have blocks. Block A, Block B, Block C …”

“Like a prison,” I said.

What I still don’t know, if I am truly honest, is what the difference is between the *Seitenflügel* and the *Quergebäude.* I know the *Hinterhaus* is opposite the *Vorderhaus,* and I know the *Seitenflügel* is connected somehow with the *Quergebäude.* And I think houses that only have one extra house only have a *Seitenflügel,* but not a *Quergebäude.* But I am not sure. I might have this all wrong. Maybe *Quergebäude* really is just another word for *Hinterhaus,* as my German editor says.* Also, this *Quergebäude* stuff confuses EVERYONE, not just foreigners. Even proper Germans. PROPER Germans. Actual Germans. If you ever get visited by an actual proper German, who wasn’t born in Berlin and only moved here a month or so ago, they’ll be as confused and bemused by the *Quergebäude* stuff as a non-German. It’s just a thing Berliners invented to make life harder for everyone. They’re good at that.**

* He’s right. — German editor

** A Twitter follower wrote to me recently and explained that there are actually secret signs posted on the houses, which I had spent twenty years blithely ignoring, with arrows on them, showing you which way the house numbers are going. Don’t wander about in the dark Berlin streets for twenty years like I did, look for the secret signs.

Chapter Eighteen:

R is for ...

Romantik: *The German word* Romantik *can mean different things in German. First up, romance, the same it means for us. Pink hearts, perfume, cuddly teddy bears. Second up, how romantic a guy is (we normally mean guys, right, because all women are romantic). How pink the pink hearts he paints you are, how expensive the perfume, how cuddly the teddy bears are. Does he take you on a weekend to Paris or does he prefer you know, a cheap getaway to Dessau or somewhere. But third, and probably most importantly, up:* gefühlsbetont.

German Romance: Not a Paradox, After All

When you first arrive in Germany, you think German boys are unromantic, of course. This is because they do these cold, sensible, unromantic, practical, unsentimental things that no human being with lungs and not gills in their chest should ever do ever, like ever ever ever FUCKING ever. They have two small duvets on their beds instead of one big one, and they never call you "darling" or "sweetie" or bring you a cup of tea in bed or tell you that you look beautiful and in the first six months of a relationship they have this weird habit of collecting your toothbrush and your deodorant and your hairclips and your tampons up every week and placing them in those see-through bags you need for liquids at the airport and handing this bag over to you at the beginning of your dinner date like it's contaminated goods or maybe they get you to PayPal them the 57.60 euros you owe them from dinner during a romantic getaway or maybe the romantic getaway they took you on was a Groupon offer and to be honest they kind of acted like they didn't really think of it as them "taking" you anywhere but instead you having failed at some kind of weird "are you German enough?" test and then spent the entire Deutsche Bahn journey "hilariously" nagging you for not having bought a Sparticket and showing off about how much they saved by getting a Sparticket in time and you just felt, more than anything else, totally fucking bored. Maybe.

At dinner, on said Groupon-based unromantic romantic getaway, they ask you if you could ever imagine getting married again, or, if you're still unmarried, ever getting married ever.

You're like: "Yeah, that's something I can envision."

Total blankness in their cold German eyes. TOTAL blankness. TOTAL BLANKNESS. The blankness is truly total, it's like staring into two swirling whirling empty German black holes of nothingness.

"I suppose because of the tax advantages?" they ask cautiously.

"Er, because I want to wear a beautiful white dress and look like a fucking princess and stand up in front of all my friends and family and declare in front of them that I want to love this guy I love forever and ever and ever more, obviously?"

If you want to see a German boy laugh, this is what you have to say.

After a while, though, you begin to understand that Germans can be romantic – but only with each other, and, I don't want to trigger anyone, only with white people. Sorry. This is kind of a controversial thing to say, because it's gonna offend everyone who can't see colour and it's also going to upset everyone who's non-white and pretending to themselves that they can join in with German romantic experiences but I am sorry guys, I am here to speak the truth and the truth is: German romance is WHITE. It's not just white, it's ashen. It's GREY. If you want a German boy to have romantic thoughts about you, you basically have to be white and blonde and skinny. Very very skinny. You have to be deathly pale and incredibly frail like people can't tell whether you've got cancer or have spent the past six years in an *Eckkneipe*, living exclusively off a diet of Currywurst and tobacco. You have to want to commit suicide, you have to be suicidal, you have to go to Wannsee and kill a fish with your bare hands. You throw the fish's corpse back into the lake. You say things like "Ich habe so viele Schmerzen in meiner Seele wie dieser Fisch, den ich gerade getötet habe." Then you go to steal a horse together. This is what counts as romantic in Germany: you have to be white, you have to be skinny, you have to be prepared to steal horses while dying of cancer and also thinking of suicide. And you really, really have to be white.

I don't know when I realised it, but one day I did: THE GERMANS ARE ROMANTIC! Just in a really fucked-up, depressingly bleak, so-white-it's-grey German kind of way. THAT'S WHY they hate shopping centres, you can't steal horses from them. That's why they prefer empty Brandenburg lakes to exciting wonderful brilliant *Spaßbads** full of people having fun. That's why they get so upset about Christmas being tacky and commercial. AND THAT'S WHY THEY HATE VALENTINE'S DAY.

* "Spaßbäder" is the correct plural. — German editor

German romance isn't actually an oxymoron, and yet still: Germans not actually finding Valentine's Day romantic is a bit of a paradox. They don't find red roses romantic. They don't find candles romantic. They don't find red rose petals and champagne and candles in a bath romantic. They don't find chocolates shaped like hearts romantic. German boys won't find it romantic if you send them a bouquet of flowers at work, take them to a posh restaurant for a candlelit dinner or send them a heart emoji on WhatsApp. It's like Germans are so romantic they've gone through the whole romance thing and come out the other side. Pink and red and purple and gorgeous colours like that are not romantic for a German. Glittery hearts are not romantic. Chocolate and sexy red underwear and snuggling underneath a beautiful warm quilt are not romantic. German romance has to be white, like a cold white rock. It has to be grey, like the bleak grey sky on a January morning. It has to be Brandenburg. Like Brandenburg.

If you want to be romantic German-style, what you need to do is act like you don't even know that the day Valentine's Day even exists. Act like you get it mixed up with Mother's Day or Women's Day or something. Screw your eyes up like you're trying to vaguely remember something from the distant past and then murmur nonchalantly "Is that the American Women's Day or something?" Then, come February 15th, cover yourself in talcum powder so you look like the fucking Joker or someone, kill a fucking fish and throw the corpse in your bed, steal a thousand horses, move to a farm in Brandenburg, weep in a boat, get seaweed in your hair. There's no glitter involved. This is German romance.

Please start taking it a bit more seriously.

Chapter Nineteen: S is for …

Schwarztee: *So, the German for tea is* Tee, *but when Germans say* Tee, *they mean any kind of tea – hibiscus, cauliflower, sage, stinging nettles, kidney and bladder, relaxation, inner peace, Christmas, fennel, peppermint (gross), camomile, lavender. If you want a nice, normal cup of tea, you have to ask for* Schwarztee *which literally means black tea. There's no specific word for drinking your tea black, because that's how they drink tea over here – black, with a bit of lemon, and also, inexplicably, out of a glass cup. They also do this awful thing where they pour the boiling water into the glass cup, put a saucer on top, and place a tea-bag on top of the saucer. The first time this ever happened to me, I thought it was some kind of passive-aggressive racist attack, because the only person, surely, you would ever do this to is someone you really hated, like hate-crime level hate? But that's just how they drink tea over here.*

When Will I Will I Be German

My stepmum, just arrived from the airport, says to me: "You've got tea in, right?"

So the most German thing I ever said was just after the Christmas market attack in 2016. I went back to the UK the next day, and the British news channels were all gloating about it – gloating is not exaggerating – and concern-trolling Germany about freedom of movement – and quoting AfD politicians as if they were "many voices in Germany".

"A sombre day in the German capital," the sad voice said, "as many Germans are waking up to the idea that everything they hold so dear – the freedom of movement within Europe – must be brought into question."

"What a load of shite!" I shouted at the screen. "When some terrorist travels from Wales to London do you guys bring anything into question?"

"Angela Merkel will be doing a lot of soul-searching tonight," the announcer said.

"She'll be doing nothing of the sort!" I yelled. "She'll be watching Netflix and having a nice bath! Angela Merkel is feeling just fine. The guy had a fake passport ANYWAY! What are they on about?"

"You're very loyal to Angela Merkel," my mum said.

"I am not," I said crossly. "I don't even like her."

"You're very loyal to the German nation," my mum said.

"I AM NOT!" I shouted. "I am loyal to the CONCEPT of Europe!""

Oh fuck, I thought, that's the most Germanest thing that ever came out of my mouth ...

NOW, looking at my stepmum, I say the second most German thing I've ever said: "I have so much tea in!" I say cheerfully. "I've got camomile, peppermint, red orange, apple, cinnamon chimney vibes, fennel and aniseed and look, this peach one. And this relaxation one. It helps you relax."

My stepmother looks at me, pure panic on her face.

"I want tea-tea!" she says.

"A nice cup of tea," my dad says.

"A nice normal cup of tea", my stepmum says. There is some judgement in her normal.

You know when you're on MDMA and your whole life swirls around you in one go and then everything falls – PLOP – back into place, but you feel like, just for one second, you'll never really be the same person again? That's this moment. When did I stop drinking black tea? When did I stop? When did I change? What happened?

I start putting my trainers on in the hall. "I'll go to the Späti," I say. "The corner shop."

"And Cint!" my dad calls from the kitchen.

"Yeah?" I say.

"Don't forget milk," he says politely.

I nod. My dad thinks I am the kind of person you have to remind to buy milk for tea now. And I guess he's right.

* * *

Shoppen versus Einkaufen: *There are two words for shopping in German,* Shoppen, *which is what you do if you're Paris Hilton, at* Galeries Lafayette, *with a credit card, looking for chanel handbags or I dunno, Manalos or something – and* Einkaufen, *which is what I do in* Lidl, *shuffling around in jogging pants, sadly looking for the cheapest yoghurt.*

Don't get Shoppen *mixed up with* Frühschoppen *though – which is a cheeky (alcoholic) drink in the morning, but not in a grimy way!*

Germans Hate Shopping Centres More Than I Hate Remoulade

"Why do Germans hate shopping centres so much?" I ask my friend Lola, as we stroll through *Neukölln Arkaden*. Maybe stroll is the wrong word. We're not doing this in a strolling, relaxing,

Shopping-Erlebnis type way. We're doing this in a hungover, headachey, slightly pukey, we-need-to-buy-eggs kind of way.

"Do they hate shopping centres?" she asks me.

"Totally!" I yell. "Think about it. Have you ever met a German who admitted that they liked a shopping centre to you?"

Lola shrugs nonchalantly. "I don't know anyone who likes shopping centres," she says softly.

"Germans hate shopping centres," I say to her. "They never admit to going to a shopping centre, ever, even when they live next door to one and there's an Aldi inside. The only Germans who admit they like shopping centres are, like, teenagers and stuff. They love shopping centres. They can shelter from the rain in them and also go shoplifting and stuff."

"But this shopping centre is full of Germans!" Lola whispers at me. "I think, like, half of the people in here are actually German."

"Hmmmn," I say. I have to admit she seems to have a bit of a point here. We are surrounded by actual Germans, and a lot of them are even white.

"My teenager loves shopping centres," I say. "Ryan is always hanging out at Gropius Passagen or Alexa. I don't need to track him like an American mum. If he ever gets in late from school I know he's gone to a shopping centre."

Lola looks at me, a bit shamefacedly. "I think, er, you know, Jacinta. I think nobody likes shopping centres."

"You think it's a Berlin thing?" I ask. "Maybe it's a Berlin thing, and I never noticed. Intellectual German Berliners hate shopping centres – but so do intellectual international Berliners. They're too intellectual to go to an optician's and a bookshop in one go. Like that would make their lives too easy or something?"

"I think, to be honest, it's a cool person thing, Jacinta," she says, and she looks a bit embarrassed to be saying it out loud.

I guess I'll just never be cool enough. I never noticed. I literally thought it was a German thing. I can still remember the weekend they built the Ilford Exchange, I'd been at my dad's for the weekend and on the Sunday, when he drove me home, we couldn't drive down the high street. The signs were this avocado green with the words Ilford Exchange kind of modern in a lumpy, 1980s way – they're still the same signs, the green has faded so much now they look kind of browny-yellow. I like shopping centres, I don't know if like isn't too strong a word. I go to them all the time and I find them perfectly fine. I enjoy shopping there. I like going to a supermarket and then to a DM.

I know why, though, I always thought it was only Germans who hated them. It was because of my German friend Jens. I remember one time I went to *Alexa* to have dinner with my son after school. I had sushi and he had *MaccyD's* and we sat in the middle bit together – this is the nice thing about eating out at Alexa, this and the fact that it's so loud there nobody comes up to you and asks you to get your kid to quieten down – and while I was waiting for my son to arrive, my German friend Jens phoned me up.

"Oh hi. I'm in Alexa," I said into my phone.

"What on earth are you doing there?" he asked, genuinely shocked.

"Eating dinner," I said.

"You poor thing," he said. "I feel so sorry for you. I assume you let Ryan choose where you'd eat tonight. God. How horrible!"

"No, I er. I wanted to come here. I wanted to have sushi and he wanted to have *McDonald's*. So that's what we do, we eat in Alexa, in the middle bit."

SILENCE. Like one of those long, cold, disapproving German silences. I think he would've been less shocked had I said

I wanted to eat dogshit scraped off of a Friedrichshain pavement.

And I think British people my age and older never hate shopping centres. We remember what there was before shopping centres – markets and stuff, yuck. When my parents visit Berlin, we have to do a tour of all their favourite Berlin shopping centres. We start off at *Potsdamer Platz Arkaden*, then go to *Neukölln-Arkaden*, then finish up at *Ring Center 1* and *2* for some Chinese noodles. They love those cheap, greasy Chinese noodles you can get in the basement of a shopping centre, they sit there, eating as slowly as possible, and every two minutes shouting to each other about how delicious but cheap it is, and how big the portions, and how much it would probably cost in Britain. Sometimes, on the way home, we pop into *Alexa*. I haven't told them about the *Mall of Berlin* yet. Or that orange monstrosity across from Warschauer Straße, *EastSide Mall* or whatever it's called.

"Actually, the other day I walked past EastSide Mall," I say to Lola as we walk round the Neukölln Kaufland. Even people who hate shopping centres must love this Kaufland. It is the best Kaufland in the world, I literally love it here. I am feeling quite hungover though, I feel like I might puke, maybe Lola's horrifically decadent idea of getting a taxi back home isn't so bad after all.

"And I thought the following words to myself. You know what I thought? 'That mall is so *unnötig*. It is a seriously *unnötig* mall.'"

"What does *unnötig* mean?" Lola asks.

"Unnecessary," I say. "And then I thought OH MY GOD I AM SO GERMAN NOW!"

Lola drops a box of eggs on the floor, and we move away quickly, as if the broken eggs have nothing to do with us. In literally any other Kaufland in Germany, broken eggs on the floor would be incredibly embarrassing, but this is the best Kaufland in Germany and the staff are just glad if you don't start masturbating over the lettuces.

"But maybe it has nothing to do with being German," I say, steering the trolley round the corner to the tills. "Maybe in my old age I am getting cool. Huh?"

Lola doesn't say anything. Perhaps she's a bit intimidated by having such a cool, older, almost-German friend, I say to myself and quickly throw a Bifi in the trolley. You're never too hungover for a Bifi.

* * *

Silvester: Silvester *is the German word for New Year's Eve. Some people spell it* Sylvester, *but it's actually* Silvester. *People can get a bit snobby about this, and usually I hate language snobbery, but to be honest, I feel like this is, in this case, a tiny bit justified: it was named after a Pope and not Sylvester Stallone, after all.*

A really good thing about German is in the run up to New Year's Eve you wish everyone a good "Rutsch" *– a nice slide – into the new year. Then after we enter the new year it's all Happy New Year* Frohes neues Jahr! *I feel like it's a bit confusing in English because in a way we start wishing everyone a happy new year from the beginning of December onwards.*

I never know from what point onwards you're not meant to say Frohes Neues *to the people who work in shops anymore, but I tend to stop around 5th January, which is my sister's birthday, and also the day in Britain when you're meant to take your Christmas decorations down.*

I Am Scared of Silvester Fireworks AND GERMANS AREN'T

"Is it true what they say about New Year's Eve in Berlin?" people who haven't been here for Silvester yet ask you sometimes. "It can't be as bad as they say it it, can it? They must be exaggerating a little? How bad can it be? They make it sound like the city turns into a war zone!"

Gather round the fireplace, newbies to Berlin, while this old wizened crone who has lived in this cold, dark city some twenty winters will let you know, in the voice of the witch from *Robin Hood: Prince of Thieves* when she sees her own death: WHATEVER YOU HAVE HEARD MY CHILDREN, THE REALITY IS EVEN WORSE!

War zone doesn't begin to cover it. Teenagers stand on balconies and merrily hurl burning missiles at your head. Every time you yelp, petrified your baby might get hurt or killed or I dunno BLINDED, the same old grannies who told you off for leaving the house in summer without putting socks on him grin at your fear nonchalantly. The said (evil) teenagers literally laugh because they know you are scared of dying and they consider this kind of emotion hugely pussyish. Your Russian best friend sighs, bored. All around you fireworks are exploding, you are literally jumping about dodging death like you're in a video game, your kids cry, dogs moan, YOUR RUSSIAN BEST FRIEND IS BORED, like she is literally bored, that's how hard she is (as nails).

"Jorcintorrrrrr," she drawls, unperturbed, unconcerned, indifferent, TOTALLY FUCKING RELAXED, "why are you so worried? German fireworks are the best in the world?"

"OLGA!" you scream. Literally all around you, everything is on fire and it is raining actual fireworks and nobody but you cares and the kids are about to die. "GOOD FIREWORKS KILL

PEOPLE! THEY ARE LITERALLY FLAMING BALLS OF FIRE THAT IS WHAT A FIREWORK IS! WHAT IS YOUR FUCKING PROBLEM?"

Your German friend, who all year long corrects her daughter's grammar, doesn't let her eat chocolate, bans Peppa Pig and Disney and Barbie because you know, sensory overload, and only lets her play with wooden toys because the chemicals in plastic apparently might damage her development or something, arrives and promptly hands all the tiny children in the vicinity BIG FUCK-OFF FIREWORKS and lets them all light them and hurl them at each other like they're fucking frisbees. You take the firework off of your kid and he starts crying, your German non-Disney watching mum friend looks at you disapprovingly.

"Do you really want to pass on your fear of fire to him, Jacinta, like Muslim women do with swimming and dogs?"

"YES!" you scream. "YES! I WANT HIM TO BE SCARED OF FIRE! BECAUSE I WANT TO GIVE HIM THE GIFT OF LIFE!"

It is literally worse than anything you have ever imagined. The next day, over breakfast, your German mum friend will be correcting her kid for saying *wegen dem* instead of *wegen des* and your Russian friend will read you the news smugly and say, "See, nobody died. Only one kid in Brandenburg got blinded and one kid in Pankow lost a hand, Jacinta. You were panicking about nothing." You just stare at her and don't speak. What is there to say? I would literally, if I could, vote Green if they introduced a fireworks ban. Some of the things I do for Greta cost me dearly (well, if I did them they would) but *Verzicht auf* Fireworks? That would come easily to me. Unfortunately, Berliners might love Greta – but they love nearly dying on Silvester more.

* * *

Späti: *The first word any newbie to Berlin learns! A* Späti *is a late-night corner shop, selling beer and tampons,* H-Milch *and cigarettes.*

The Poshest Späti in Town

A friend of mine lives in Kreuzberg and the Späti next to her house is so posh they sell almond milk, oat milk AND soya milk. I live in Lichtenrade and we don't have any Spätis – at night, we have to go to the *Tankstelle* and order food (or, let's be honest, drink) at the emergency counter. On a Sunday, we can do bakeries, or said *Tankstelle* – but if you need nappies you have to go to Südkreuz or an emergency chemist. It's literally like living in some kind of dystopian nightmare.

The only good thing about living in Lichtenrade – well apart from the fact that my rent is affordable and there are actually flats here which ordinary people can live in – is that the Dönerläden all sell beer, Sekt, and tiny cans of vodka mixed with lemonade. Who needs oat milk when you can wash your Dönerfleisch down with swigs of sickly alcohol? But if you want to go out for a nice relaxing Sunday brunch, you literally have to go to a bakery like a Rentner, or get on the fucking U-Bahn.

As Berlin gets more and more gentrified, and the rents get higher and higher – like, nothing surprises me anymore, like someone can literally tell me "They're renting out luxury mini-apartments in Marzahn for 2500 euros a month, which are actually just beds in a cupboard and the kitchen sink is actually in the shower" and I shrug nonchalantly – and as the few friends I have who are actually happy and married (puke) keep on moving to the suburbs, or even, in some cases, the countryside, I keep on trying to kid myself that I actually want to live here, and sometimes it almost works. But the truth is, I want to live somewhere where the Spätis sell weird milk, and I buy normal milk, and everyone looks down on me for it. It's kind of a nice feeling, being one of the boring ones. I'm definitely not boring for Lichtenrade. I'm the most interesting person who ever set foot here.

* * *

Spielplatz: Spiel *means play and* Platz *means place. Put them together and what have you got? A playground!* Kinderspielplatz *means a children's playground. Berlin playgrounds are a million times better than the ones I grew up "playing" on which were so boring I think Isis wouldn't even have bothered banning them.*

Berlin Playground Etiquette

Berlin playgrounds are great, in my eyes. I am totally Berlin about this, I feel super-patriotically proud of them. They are brilliant. I was about seven years old when all the proper see-saws in Britain got replaced with dinky little bouncy things that didn't actually go click, click, clickety-clack, see-saw, see-saw, but just rubbishly bobbed up and down on separate bouncy springs. Going to a Berlin playground is just this glorious experience for me. Proper see-saws! Proper wooden climbing frames stretching high into the sky that your kid could easily fall off the top of, landing on the ground with a huge thwack, breaking every bone in their body. All that sand. Oh, the joy of being a Berlin parent, sitting at the side of the playground, being handed a cone of sandy "ice-cream".

"Is that for me?" You ask, even though you know it is.

"Yummy," says your toddler gravely.

"Is it yummy?" you ask.

"A yummy ice-cream for Mummy?"

"Dorbry," says your toddler, which is, as you know, in toddlerspeak, the correct word for strawberry. Berlin playgrounds are glorious. They are wonderful. They are magnificent. Nobody loves them more than me.

The only problem with Berlin playgrounds? All the bloody *Ausländer*, and I say *Ausländer*, but if I am truly honest, I mean Americans, who don't know the playground etiquette. There's playground etiquette. There's social norms to be followed. There's rules to be obeyed:

1. DO NOT GREET THE OTHER PARENTS

Germans love to greet each other for no reason at all, like total inexplicable greetings are mandatory here – *but weirdly not at the playground!* Sometimes when I have been in the UK a while, I come back to Germany and I greet everyone at the playground, like you do here at the doctor's – and everyone shoots me puzzled glances like I am slightly mad. Don't greet other parents at the playground. I don't know why, but it just isn't done.

2. SHARE FOOD – BUT ONLY *BIO* PLEASE!

So I don't actually like to give my kid grapes all day long, I don't really think he needs to be grazing and grazing and grazing like a fucking cow munching on grass ... BUT I have to bring a tupperware box filled with the most boring toddler food possible – grapes, boring rice cakes, tiny cheese *Stanges*, the kind of stuff nobody wants to eat, just so when your kid has been panhandling from strangers all afternoon, you can give their kids some grapes back and avoid actually dying of actual shame. I know from an American friend that this isn't the done thing in America, where everyone is worried about food allergies and getting sued and stuff. But it is totally socially acceptable here, and in fact refusing food too brusquely seems a bit rude. However, the food has to be healthy, *bio* – and boring as fuck. My mother lived in a really multicultural part of East London, where mums in headscarves rock on up to the playground, greet everyone, and unpack an unhealthy picnic full of stuff that no Berlin mum would ever eat ever – chocolate fingers, sponge cakes, salt and vinegar crisps. They then hand the food out in the manner of Jesus feeding the five thousand. A lot of the mums expect you to take half the food home. Last summer, I actually asked a Bangladeshi mum I met at the playground: "Why are you giving me this?" I was worried she thought we were poor or something. She looked at me knowingly, lovingly, reassuringly and whispered: "It's nice to share."

3. SHARING IS CARING: OKAY, YOU DON'T NEED TO FORCE YOUR KID TO FUCKING SHARE – BUT DON'T BE A DICK ABOUT IT

Look, Americans. You go to the fucking playground. IT IS A COMMUNAL FUCKING PLAYSPACE. No, you don't have to "force" your darling kid to "share" his precious sandpit toys (cheapo plastic crap from China that is worth about 50 cents max, let's be honest). However, you should expect your kids to share, and you should tell them that the playground is a public space, and you should tell them that the toys they bring to the playground are for everyone to use and when you go home, you'll get them back. YES EVEN THE BOBBY-CARS AND BALANCE BIKES. It's so mad to see these American mothers at the playground, frantically chasing some toddler around because said toddler is playing with a plastic digger and said plastic digger actually belongs to her baby.

An American friend of mine once said she wouldn't force her kid to share playground toys because she doesn't share her mobile phone with the other parents at the playground. Okay, let's get down to this. Actually, yes, if someone NEEDED your phone, you would fucking share it – because you are a human being and not a sociopath and the achievement of having paid money to own something doesn't trump your duty as a human being to help another person who needs to borrow your phone for two seconds. But, secondly, the analogy is all wrong. Not sharing your playground toys at the playground is the equivalent of meeting up for a barbecue and not sharing the fucking barbecue because it's "yours" or meeting up for a game of badminton but the badminton rackets are all yours and so now you're not going to play any badminton because you're not willing to share. If you really think that your children will be so traumatised and scarred by the idea that playground toys, for the duration of the playground visit, belong to everyone, why not stay at fucking home and leave everyone else in fucking peace.

The other thing is, you don't need to "force" them to share. Nobody needs to "force" their kid to share. You just explain to them, like a fucking PARENT. Sometimes you'll use his spade, sometimes she'll use your digger, look here, sometimes we can use this cone. You're not using it right now, so it makes sense for this kid to use it. And if you share, you can play together and have this totally-alien-concept-to-American-parents-obviously thing called fun with each other.

4. IT IS ABSOLUTELY FINE TO NICK A SANDCASTLE BUCKET FROM THE PLAYGROUND IF IT HAS BEEN LEFT THERE FOR, LIKE, OVER TWO WEEKS

Really don't understand why anyone ever pays for sandpit toys to be honest.

5. KIDS GET NAKED GET OVER IT

Just let them be kids and stop going on about paedos. They're kids, for Christ's sake. To quote my ex-mother-in-law: "Isn't that the nicest thing about being a child? Spending the whole summer naked in the playground?"

6. SLIDE ETIQUETTE

Okay, so it is absolutely fine for your kid to go UP the slide IF there are no other kids in the park. It is kind of okay for your kid to go up the slide if all the other kids are also going up the slide too, though some pussy German mums will get annoyed by this behaviour. It is not okay for your kid to go up the slide if there is a queue of kids waiting to slide down. It is kind of okay for your kid to be super-brave and think they can handle this slide, then mount the top and chicken out and sit there, causing a Stau. It really is kind of okay, it's good for kids to be brave. But don't let them cause a *Stau* for longer than 2.5 minutes. After 2.5 minutes, you need to persuade your kid to get sliding – or even get up there yourself and drag him down yourself.

7. PARK-TIME IS PHONE-TIME

The whole point of going to the playground is to ignore your child as much as possible, let them enjoy their independent playtime, connect with other children, and you play Wordblitz/2048/get Instagramming. I say this as someone whose child once tried to lorry their way down concrete steps while I had, wonderfully, tantalisingly, beautifully, 1024 on two separate squares on either side of my 2048 block. He didn't die. They're meant to play with other kids.

8. FLIRT WITH THE DADS

Every now and then, some dad will do some "woe is me" victim mentality mindset column about how isolated they are at the playground, where all the mums are in one corner swapping breastfeeding tips and rubbing their pregnant bellies with lavender oils and shooting hateful glances at the dad like he shouldn't even be there but out at Siemens/IBM/some startup. Don't let the dicks get away with this. It's your duty to flirt as outrageously as possible with the one dad at the playground. We need those woe-is-me-victim-mentality-isolated-dad-at-the-playground articles to be a bit more interesting in the future.

* * *

Steile These: *Hot take, though Germans, being cleverer than us, all know what hot takes are too.*

Heisses Nehmen

"A hot take is a *steile These* in German," I tell my teenage boy.

"Wow, that's a bit of a hot take!" he says, almost mockingly.

"You know I'm right," I say.

"It's a warmish take at least," he says.

"A slightly sloping theory," I say.

"Oh God, shut up!" he says and I walk away. I know I'm right.

Bonus Chapter: ß is for …

S-Zett: *One time, when we went back to the UK, my son was about five or six years old. Our family was super full, my mum still alive, and my brother and sister home, too. My mum must have been able-bodied enough, still, to make it out into the kitchen – in later years her MS stopped her doing this. We sat in the kitchen, everyone talking to each other and over each other, as families are wont to do. My son, who hadn't been speaking at all, pulled me by the hand into the living room. He wanted to speak to me alone.*

"Mum," he said. "In English I don't need to say the T in words."

I was surprised by his statement. But I agreed with it, and didn't bother specifying that not everyone in England would agree with him.

"No," I said. "You can leave it out."

"But not at the beginning of words," he said.

I was really surprised by this. I had literally never thought of it before.

"No," I agreed.

"It's Wha'," he said, pronouncing the word what in the perfect cockney way.

"Yeah," I said. "When you're in England, you can say it like that."

"But it's still table," he said carefully. "Not 'able."

"No," I said.

He bounced away from me cheerfully and sat himself down at the table, and shouted boisterously: "Nana, I wan' wa'er!"

This is probably where the similarities between the glottal stop and the S-Zett *end but: never start a word with one.* Das geht nicht!

Snakey B

S-Zett, or, to give it its official name, "that weird snaky German B letter" is probably the most fun, exciting thing about being able to speak – or write, actually – German. IT'S SO MUCH FUN. A New York friend of mine, named Strauss, told me Straub is a really common surname in New York – and we all know why. It's the same reason as why my parents used to send my letters to Flughafenstrabe. IT'S BECAUSE IT'S A WHOLE ENTIRE LETTER WE DON'T HAVE IN ENGLISH!

I guess you noticed that we don't have it in English? Guess what, though? They don't have it in Swiss German either. God the ß is cool. It's literally the coolest letter ever.

It stands for a double S – but, annoyingly, you don't need it half the time. You need it in *Straße* but not in *Hass* – I guess the rule is, like, is the vowel beforehand long or short?

WRITING THEM IS SO MUCH FUN. THEY ARE THE MOST FUN THING IN THE GERMAN LANGUAGE EVER, POSSIBLY IN THE WHOLE WORLD, ACTUALLY PROBABLY IN THE WHOLE UNIVERSE. So much fun. They just flow so easily off of your pen, like the slinky, dinky, drunken, cheeky Weimar Republic caterpillars that they are (note to people who actually care about these things, of course they are actually ages old and loads older than the Weimar Republic, but they also give off a very dinky and cute, old-fashioned in a modern way, kind of a vibe). If you ever meet a potential partner with an ß in their surname, if you are a feminist chick you will throw all your feminist ideals out the window, if you are a sexist bloke, you'll discover your inner male feminist, and if you are a nonbinary genderfluid type person, you won't worry about this stuff, AND MARRY THEM IMMEDIATELY, taking their surname and embracing happineß for the rest of your life. The beautiful, perfect, delicious, wonderful S-Zett. So much fun. The S-Zett, alone, is worth moving to Germany for.

Chapter Twenty: T is for ...

Theater: Theater *means theatre, but it also means making a fuss about things, being melodramatic, causing a scene ...*

The Good Thing About German Theatre

My ex-in-laws are not the most, erm, what shall we say, open-minded of people? I love them and they (I think) love me, but they are very, very, very German. I once told my ex mother-in-law that we didn't put sugar in English potato salad and she just shut me down completely. "Potato salad", she said resolutely, like kids, when they've just found out about the Earth going round the sun, "has one teaspoon of sugar in it."

I honestly think that my ex married me to piss his parents off, but you know what it's like. His parents, if I am ever back on Hartz IV, will literally slag refugees off to my face and then say "And you poor thing have to pay your child benefit back to the job centre! What is this country coming to – all the money in the world for refugees but none for our own people?"

Our own people – *unsere eigenen Leute*. And it only took me marrying their son, giving them a grandchild, having two kids in Germany and living here for one million years. There is hope for all of us!

“We were really worried for a while,” my ex father-in-law says. They've come over for a bit of coffee and cake in my living room, before driving on to see my ex.

“Oh,” I say.

“There was an English man who got the job as the boss of our nearest opera! You can imagine how worried we were. A foreigner.”

My son hides a smile while I nod tactfully/hypocritically.

“Yes,” I say.

I don't bother arguing because I think it's better I save all my energy for sticking up for actual refugees and people like that – English expats running operas can stick up for themselves, I figure.

“But do you know? He's doing a lovely job.”

“Lovely.”

“Just perfect.”

“They wear costumes from the times the opera is set in, it's so nice.”

“No dead animals on the stage.”

“They never smash anything up for no reason.”

“And no nudity!”

“Nice costumes, sensible props, and everything just kind of ... fits together somehow.”

“Going to the opera has never been so much fun!”

“I'm glad,” I say.

Me, personally, I like the German way of doing theatre or operas. I like it. You go, and you concentrate, and you try really hard. The weird thing is, you have to concentrate just as much on stuff you know the plot to – “Emilia Galotti” or “Woyzeck” – as stuff you've never heard before. You get a bit of a headache from all the concentrating. And JUST AT THE POINT when you think you literally cannot concentrate for one second more, they either a) get out a dead animal and start cutting it up b) get naked c) smash the stage up or d) do all three. Then you get a little break from concentrating on hard German words, because obviously you can't do that at the same time as looking at strangers' willies and boobies, can you. At the exact point your brain has recovered from all the German language concentration, they put their clothes on and get back to the story.

The only trouble is, it does mean you can't actually remember the plots of any German *Klassiker*. Conversations about German classic plays you've seen always always always go like this:

"Jacinta, have you seen 'Kabale und Liebe'?"

"Yes, that's the one where they smash the stage up, right?"

"Jacinta, did you ever see 'Faust'?"

"Yes, they sliced up a dead pig after about two hours, right?"

"Jacinta, you seen 'Die Räuber'."

"Oh absolutely. Will never forget it. Lovely boobs, but one of them had such a weird penis."

I've never really understood why the same people who act like the world is ending when kids' classic books get slightly updated texts so that they're, you know, slightly easier for young children to understand, don't mind everyone walking about naked with lamb smeared across their faces and smashed up chairs burning across the stage when it comes to the theatre. But there you go. There are some things about Germany, quite simply, that are a little bit hard to understand. And by some things I mean quite literally everything they do and say.

* * *

Toastbrot: Toastbrot *means sliced bread you CAN toast – the* Toastbrot *you buy in Germany is all shit – Sammy's Sandwich Toast, sage ich nur. Germans have not realised you can put any bread in the toaster if you slice it thin enough.*

Brot – *pronounced BROOOOOOOOOOOOOOOT – is normally* Schwarzbrot – *kind of yummy, in an earthy, woody way, but it is a bit like eating cement. I once wrote "bread" on the shopping list instead of "Toastbrot" and my son came back with proper German bread, BROOOOOOOOOOOOOT, all wrapped up in posh waxy paper and everything.*

"Oh," I said, strangely pleased. "Proper German bread! Why didn't you buy the bread we normally get?"

"Because that's not bread!" my son said. "It's toast bread!"

"Let's eat some now," I say.

"I'm not going to EAT that! I'm a kid. Kids eat Schrippen*" – plain white rolls – "or toast."*

"Why did you buy bread you don't want to eat?"

"You put it on the list," he said, shrugging nonchalantly.

I've never spent so much time on the toilet as I did that week – no wonder German women are so skinny, they must be shitting their entire body weight out in Kacke *every week.*

Ungetoastetes Toastbrot

"Jacinta," my German friend writes me on Facebook. "Wie sagt man ungetoastetes Toastbrot auf Englisch?" (How do you say untoasted sliced bread in English?)

I write back: "Bread."

He writes back: "HA HA HA!"

I write back nothing.

He writes back: "You're a very funny person, one of the funniest people I know, but seriously now, just answer the question."

I write back: "BREAD."

He writes back: "I'm not stupid."

I think to myself: "You're not stupid, you're just German."

The thing about the whole Toastbrot situation which I don't quite get is that nobody forced the Germans to make their Toastbrot that shit. Bread in the UK is bad, yeah, worse than bread in Germany, sure – but the Toastbrot in the UK is much better than Toastbrot in Germany, and not that much worse than the normal bread you buy in plastic at the supermarket, rather than the baker's counter. In fact, our most expensive Toastbrot must be better than the cheapest sliced bread non-Toastbrot in Germany? My son once ate a whole loaf of Kingsmill at my granddad's house in one go. He just sat there and kept on saying yes whenever my granddad offered him another slice – until, eventually, the whole packet was gone.

I feel sorry for Germans in London who miss their proper German bread – but I miss crumpets more, I think. The butter oozing down the holes – the sogginess mixed with the crispness and the butteriness – all mixed together into one heavenly perfectionness. They keep on opening up new hipster bars in Neukölln – porridge and haggis and fish and chips and roast dinners are taking over all the old *Eckkneipen*. Let me know when the first crumpet bar opens up. I'll be there faster than you can say: "Ungetoastetes Toastbrot auf Englisch heißt einfach Bread."

Chapter Twenty-One: U is for ...

Umlaut: *Okay so watch out. What we think* Umlauts[*] *are – lovely dots with which you can randomly decorate words as you see fit – are not, in the German world,* Umlauts *at all.*

Umlauts *are important to Germans. For example: back home in East London,* Umlauts *are in. As decoration. There's a video games shop near my mum's house called Fün Shop. My teenage son always explains to me that this means it should actually be pronounced in a Northern accent. Foooon shop. I don't think there are any British people who agree with him, including, I suspect, all the German teachers and professors in the country. British people are just genetically incapable of caring about* Umlauts.

Or what about the two dots on top of the E in Zoë? As my friend Fabian is always telling me, they're nice and all, but they're not Umlauts! The German Umlauts *are something really special indeed.*

There's ä as in Änderungen.

There's ö as in Öl.

And there's ü as in Überwinden.

A terrible secret about me is that I hear Umlauts *where there aren't any. Twenty years here, and I think the German politician Wolfgang Kubicki's*[**] *name sounds like it should be pronounced*

---

* Correct German plural is "Umlaute". — German editor

** Sexy but annoying Liberal who spent the whole of Lockdown drinking cocktails at an illegal pub, but he's such a silver fox he gets away with everything.

Kübicki. I blame my Essex accent. I pronounce room roooooooooooo-ooooooooo-um.

Unnecessary Umlauts

"Mum, this absence note you've written me for school is just full of unnecessary Umlauts. Like, every single Umlaut you've put on is unnecessary and the only word which actually needed an Umlaut is *unumlauted*!"

"That's not a word!"

"Can you rewrite it?"

"Can you not just cross them out?"

"Please just rewrite it normally, Mum."

I'm about to remind him of how, when he was little, he used to spell the English word hurt "hört" but it's crazy early in the morning and instead I decide to just go back to bed.

"Schläf güt Jacinta," I say to myself as gorgeous sleep washes all over me.

* * *

Unzuverlässig: *There's no real German word for flakey – but* unzuverlässig *means unreliable. Reliable, therefore, is* zuverlässig. *To rely on someone is:* Ich verlasse mich auf dich.

Germans Can Be Surprisingly Flakey Sometimes!

So this is what happens when you meet up with any nationality of person who isn't a German, anyone, and I literally mean ANYONE: Hungarian, Mongolian, American, Thai, Russian, Spanish and/or Israeli, but of course, most of all, British:

1. You make a vague plan on Facebook chat three weeks in advance.

2. You make a slightly less vague plan on Facebook chat two weeks in advance.

3. One week to go! The vague plan is totally changed – if you were going to go swimming, you will now go to the theatre. If you wanted to go to the opera, you will now go to see *James Bond* at *Babylon*. If you were planning on hanging out in a park and drinking cider, you will now go and hang out by the canal with a bottle of Rotkäppchen.

4. Two days before said meeting: one thousand Facebook chat messages confirming that everything is "still on" and "all good" and "we're still set for tomorrow."

5. IT'S THE DAY OF THE *VERABREDUNG*! Now you switch to WhatsApp and send each other 74,000 messages deciding where to meet, when to meet, who is buying the tickets, and checking that you wouldn't actually ACTUALLY prefer to just come over for coffee instead.

6. Twenty minutes before *Verabredung*: obligatory WhatsApp message explaining that you're running late, is the person you're meeting running late too?

7. WhatsApp, WhatsApp, WhatsApp, WhatsApp. I will meet you by the kiosk with the blow-up dolphin in the window. There's no kiosk with a blow-up dolphin in the window? Maybe they took the blow-up dolphin out of the window of said kiosk. Okay, shall we meet at the other kiosk. You know the other kiosk. The one where we met up with Spanish Paul that time and he pretended he'd just eaten a pigeon for breakfast. Oh no maybe we should just meet on the platform after all. Oh, fuck, *Schienenersatzverkehr* ... Schienenersatzverkehr, in other words: I SHOULD BE ON A TRAIN ACTUALLY GETTING SOMEWHERE BUT INSTEAD I AM ON A BUS A SLOW BUS A SLOOOOOOOOOW BUS INCHING ITS WAY SLOW-

LY SLOWLY SLOOOOOOOWLY THROUGH BERLIN EVERYONE ON THE BUS IS POOR I DON'T MEAN THAT IN A JUDGY WAY NOBODY ON THIS BUS HAS EVER WORKED EVER I HATE POORSHAMING ACTUALLY BUT I AM ON A BUS WITH POOR PEOPLE WHEN I SHOULD BE ON A TRAIN AND I HATE MY LIFE.

8. Twenty minutes after planned *Verabredung* was meant to commence one final WhatsApp message deciding that you will meet directly at venue.

9. You finally meet, hurrah!

10. You are so fucking exhausted from the stress of meeting up with people with this kind of military planning – like seriously, Hitler put less effort into strategically invading France in 1940 than you just have in meeting up for drinks – that you can't even tell if you're actually having fun or not. You suspect you might be.

THIS IS HOW (ESPECIALLY WHITE BUT BASICALLY ALL OF 'EM) GERMANS MEET UP:

1. In December you make a plan to meet up in January. You decide a time and a place. You remember this time and place, because it will come in handy later.

2. IN JANUARY YOU STICK TO IT. THERE ARE NO CONFIRMATION E-MAILS. THERE ARE NO *SCHIENENERSATZVERKEHR*-BASED DISASTERS. THERE IS NO PLAN CHANGING. You said you'd be at the Siegesäule at 15:30 on January 8th, and by God you are.

Honestly, it's like Germans think the cold war is still going on, the absoluteness and constancy with which they *verabreden* themselves, using monuments and landmarks and memory – "see you there" – "it's noted in my diary" – and they bloody well will see you there too instead of WhatsApping you a million times to confirm and/or change plans. If you ever do send a confirmation text/WhatsApp message to a German, they get almost offended – "It's in my diary Jacinta, we planned it, haven't you planned it, haven't you written it down in your diary?" Kind of offended, kind of bemused, a tiny bit hurt.

It's telling, too, I always think, that there is no word in English for *verabredet* – I am meeting someone later. I am meant to be meeting someone later. Oh, I am going to meet up with a friend later. Wishy-washy, half-hearted, inconstant. I AM *VERABREDET* – and I will be there – I SAID I WILL BE THERE AND I WILL! It's set in stone. Verabredungs* are set in stone, almost in a Narnia-like way.

But this is not to say Germans can't be flakes. If you've been living here for a bit, you know. You knooooooooow. You know. They can be fucking flaky sometimes. THE FLAKIEST THINGS GERMANS DO IS WHEN THEY SAY THEY ARE NOT COMING TO YOUR BIRTHDAY PARTY BECAUSE THEY HAVE TO *INHALIEREN*! Honestly, I have literally no idea why they don't just lie and make up a good excuse, this is literally what the concept of lying was invented for: when you care so little about someone that you'd prefer to stay home and *Inhalieren* than schlep yourself to their birthday party. But still. I suppose we have to let them off here. It's stressful enough for us, meeting up with other *Ausländer*. It must drive the Germans bonkers!

* "Verabredungen" is the correct plural. — German editor

Chapter Twenty-Two: V is for ...

Verwandte: Verwandte *means relative, and it's one of those weird German words you can't make feminine. So while German speakers will say to you "Isn't it annoying when you're speaking English and someone tells you a story about a cousin and you have to stop them and ask them if it's a male or female cousin?" ACTUALLY IF THEY STOPPED TO THINK ABOUT IT FOR TWO SECONDS THEY WOULD REALISE THEY ACTUALLY HAVE A WORD THAT FUNCTIONS EXACTLY THIS WAY: in German, your female relatives are your* weibliche Verwandte *and not your* Verwandtinnen. *Other words which you can't gender up include* Gast *(some people do, though) and* Staatsoberhaupt *(the Queen of England is a* Staatsoberhaupt *and not a* Staatsoberhauptin*).**

Germans Don't Love their Relatives – They Just Like them. A LOT Though

Am sitting with a German dad at the Spielplatz and we are indulging in the German equivalent of small talk, i.e. swapping anecdotes about horrific Amt experiences, complaining about the *Senat*, and every now and then he tells me a tragic

* It's even more weird: With indefinite articles there *are* male and female forms: "ein Verwandter/eine Verwandte". I'm sorry. — German editor

DDR story, like maybe about a deaf child drowning to death in the bath tub or something. We are having about as much fun as it is humanly possible to have in a Spielplatz in Germany, basically.

My son comes up to me and gives me a plastic cup full of wet sand.

"Coffee!" He says.

"Mmmmn," I say. I make what I think are loud coffee drinking noises.

"Nicht essen!" My son says sternly. "Not ice. Coffee. Nicht essen."

"Sorry," I say.

East German dad at the Spielplatz's kid comes up to him.

"Here's some ice-cream for you," he says in perfect German. "Here you go Dad."

He also hands his dad a plastic cup of wet sand. It's kind of nice, the role reversal at the playgrounds – the kids feeding us for once – even if the thing they feed us is cold, wet sand.

"I love you Dad!" the kid says. "Ich liebe dich, Papa!"

His dad grins, and beams and kind of winces all at the same time.

"Ich liebe dich auch, Kleiner!" he whispers back and the boys run off to throw sticks in a puddle.

"This is your doing," he says to me in English once the boys have run off.

"What?" I ask.

"All this I love you stuff," he says. "It's your fault. Do you think I ever told my parents I loved them? It's all the English speakers' doing. You've turned our kids into mushy Americans! My son tells me he loves me every day!"

"You never told your parents you loved them?"

"I told them I had them lieb once a year. On my birthday!"

"I'm sorry," I say.

"Oh don't apologise," he says. "I like it. It is a bit embarrassing though. But I even say it back sometimes."

GERMANS DON'T SAY "I LOVE YOU". They have each other love – *sie haben sich lieb*. It means less than "I love you", which they really save for special occasions. The thing is, you have to realise: the English words "I love you" literally mean less than the German words *"ich liebe dich"*. Like, if you were a translator – and I am not – and you were translating someone leaving the house one morning – "Love you, Mum! See you later!" You would translate that as: "Habe dich lieb, Mama! Bis später!"

I remember once, on the balcony, my first husband's – that does, I admit, make it sound like I have 74 husbands' skeletons rotting away in the cellar – parents were leaving, and my son and I, he was about three at the time, were waving them off in their car. I whispered to my son: "Tell them you love them!" And he shouted down from the top of the balcony: "Ich habe euch ganz gern!" (To have someone *gern* is even less loving than having them *lieb*, I reckon – a good translation would be: you're kind of okay.)

But it's not just a translation issue. Remember how people in "Anne of Green Gables" books complain about the youngsters overusing the word love? Germans are like old people in "Anne of Green Gables" – they think love is hard and special and heavy and sacred. You shouldn't love vegan sausages and the glitter episode of *Peppa Pig* and Kreuzkölln on a Saturday night. You should only love people, and only people you've chosen to, and only with all your heart – and you don't need to tell them about it every two seconds.

"Does your Uncle Jens love you?" I asked my son, Ryan a few years back. "I know Germans don't tell each other they love each other. But do you think he does?"

"Oh, Mum, it's different with German relatives."

"Is it?"

"Yeah. They don't actually love you. They just like you. A LOT."

"Really?"

"In a way it's better to be liked a lot than loved a little, Mum."

"Is it?"

"It's safer."

Germany's changing now. People are saying "I love you" more often, and also that they love vegan sausages more often. Germany is changing. Social media is changing Germany, and also, in my eyes, the millions and zillions and squillions of English-speaking hipsters are changing Germany (more than the refugee wave I'd say.) Netflix is changing Germany. Non-white Germans, too, are changing Germany. C'mon it had to happen some time. They couldn't have carried on being totally German forever.

But don't be too sad if your German boyfriend hasn't told you he loves you yet. He might just be waiting. He might just be being German.

Chapter Twenty-Three: W is for …

Wachsen: *So you know how in English, flammable and inflammable mean the same thing? I can't, off the top of my head, think of any examples like this in the German language.*

What German does have though, are times when the same word can mean the opposite thing. Umfahren *is an example of this, as is* Wachsen.

Wachsen *can mean grow – you know, like how in English we talk about a waxing moon?* Wachsen *means grow, and* Erwachsen *means grown-up. People used to say Germans never said "Grow up!" as an insult – but I guess all the American movies dubbed into English have meant that people can now say "Werde erwachsen!" or even "Werde endlich mal erwachsen!" (I have heard this a few times!)*

But Wachsen *also means: to wax, as in, to wax your legs.*

And so: if the hair on your legs is wachsing too much, you need to get wachsing!

Also: don't get wachsen *mixed up with* wichsen, *which is pronounced EXACTLY like vixen, a female fox, and means to wank.* Wichser *is a wanker, and you literally never hear anyone, no matter how woke they are, saying* Wichserin.

How Does Your Garden (or Balcony) Grow?

Berlin is incomprehensibly posh now – and the exotic plants craze proves it.

A few years ago, people in Berlin liked Currywurst and drugs and literally nothing else. Currywurst and drugs. There was literally nothing else anybody living in Berlin liked doing ever except eating Currywrust and taking drugs.

Boy oh boy, how times have changed. Berlin is no longer "poor but sexy" (as former mayor Klaus Wowereit once said) – it's now kind of expensive and a bit weird. Kind of posh, in an incomprehensible way. Everyone has hobbies now, have you noticed that? It's not just Currywurst for breakfast and ketamine for dinner anymore. People have hobbies, proper hobbies, that they take seriously and do regularly. I feel so left out of this hobby craze. When did Berliners decide to get hobbies? Where was I when this hobby memo got sent out?

And, without a doubt, the weirdest hobby of all time is owing houseplants. Not just any plants, but incredibly expensive exotic plants.

"What do you think of my exotic houseplant collection?" my friend Lola asks me. I blink a bit, stare at her exotic houseplant collection – it's hard to see where her exotic houseplant collection ends and the rest of her bedroom begins to be honest – and try to think of something to say.

"Did you rob *Tropical Islands* or something?" I ask.

I haven't been over to Lola's for about a year or so – she's a druggy friend, and I have a toddler and am hence in full-on mum mode – and our paths just haven't crossed for a while. But now, here I am, in her bedroom, which was always surprisingly elegant for someone whose main dating strategy is to become all sexy German boys' unofficial drug dealer, and I might as well be in the greenhouse bit at Kew Gardens.

"Do you like this one?" she asks, pointing at a luscious spiky thing, which, you know, looks really really fucking nice. I'm not crazily into plants but you'd have to have a heart of stone not to like it. I bet even people like Donald Trump and Erdogan and Putin and people like that would feel a tiny bit of joy in their hearts when they look at this luscious spiky green thing. "Guess how much it cost?"

Oh, fuck. I wonder how much it cost. I do NOT have green thumbs, green fingers – I don't even have a green vagina. The only plants I ever buy are those shitty pots of basil from Kaufland – and they're always dead within the week. But even to my untrained eye, I can tell this was an expensive plant. It's so deliciously green and not German-looking.

"50 euros?" I take a stab in the dark.

Lola beams at me joyously.

"89 euros!" She announces grandly.

"Wow," I say. "That's a lot of money that you could've been spending on drugs or taxis."

"It's my new hobby," she explains gravely. What's happened to this city, I think to myself. What fucking happened?

Some sexy German boys come over to unofficially pick up drugs. Kai-Sebastian and Phillipp. You're not meant to call women girls anymore, but I think we're still allowed to call German boys "boys". They're something so unmanly about German males under 30, isn't there? Something desperately boyish about their shoulders, glasses and haircuts.

"I love your exotic plant collection!" Kai-Sebastian gasps with delight. "Where did you get this beauty from?" he asks, fingering a plant with big red bell-shaped petals.

"Bauhaus," says Lola, glowing with pride.

A bit of disapproval creeps into Kai-Sebastian's eyes.

"You just went to Bauhaus and bought yourself a tropical plant, just like that?"

"Yeah?" Lola says, looking worried.

"Oh," says Kai-Sebastian. "I never do that. What I do is, I get all my plants for free. I secretly take clippings from hotels or I steal them from bars and restaurants. It's a matter of pride for me. I would never be so basic," Kai-Sebastian sighs sadly "as to just go to Bauhaus and buy myself a big, expensive plant." Kai-Sebastian pauses for a moment. Lola looks completely crestfallen. "That's the kind of thing my older brother, who works in IT, would do."

AUWA! When I made my comment about robbing Tropical Islands, I thought I was being sarcastic – but Kai-Sebastian is living the dream. Lola gets out a five-euro bottle of Lidl wine for us to get chugging on. There's probably about three thousand euros' worth of luscious rainforest greenery in here, but we're still drinking wine that tastes like paint stripper. I guess in some ways, Berlin will never get posh.

* * *

Westdeutschland: *Okay so listen up you guys, things are about to get complicated.* Westdeutschland *means, obviously, West Germany.* Ostdeutschland *is East Germany. Germans don't really talk about* Westdeutschland *anymore – especially not when talking about the Western area of our country Germany. Instead, they normally specify the area they mean, the actual Bundesland (federal state). But Germans still say* Ostdeutschland *to mean both East Germany, the DDR, the GDR, the country that used to exist – and to also mean the area now, which used to be this country. It can get a bit confusing sometimes.*

People also use the former East – ehemaliger Osten – *to talk about these areas (the geographical places which exist now). They will also say "new federal states":* die neuen Bundesländer *(and I only found out recently that the* Bundesländer *Brandenburg, Thü-*

ringia, Saxony, Saxony-Anhalt, Mecklenburg-Pomerania didn't exist as administrative states in the DDR).

So Westdeutschland, *West Germany, was known as the* Bundesrepublik Deutschland *(BRD), the Federal Republic of Germany. And the country we live in today is called this too, they're the same country. East Germany, also known as the* Deutsche Demokratische Republik, *the German Democratic Republic, was essentially sucked into the BRD, you know like how the big twin will eat the little twin in the womb.*

Oh, and one nice thing people say is East Times: Ostzeiten. *I love it, like as if a geographical place can be an era of time. But I suppose it can be. I suppose it kind of is.*

My dad and my oldest boy are playing a kind of taboo game my dad has made up himself.

"This country has won the world cup four times," my son says.

"Italy," my dad says.

"No ..." my son says.

"Brazil, then."

No!" Ryan calls. "Germany!"

"Well, not really," my dad says gently. "West Germany has won it three times. But Germany today has only won once."

"You're just saying that because you're jealous!" my son calls.

"No, I'm not!" my dad says. "The Germans really deserved to win. They were a good team, that German team who won. But West Germany won three times, and united Germany has only won once. I bet people are much prouder, huh, Cint, that they won as a united country? They must have been so proud."

The way Brits talk – and think – about Germany's reunification is all, all wrong. It's sweet, and cute, but wrong. I think it's an innocent mistake – I think during the cold war, they hardly ever called West Germany the Bundesrepublik, *or the Federal State of Germany, whereas they DID call East Germany the DDR some-*

times. So they mistakenly believe that there were two countries – East Germany and West Germany – who came together at the end of communism, as communism failed, to create a new, stronger, united country: GERMANY.

*The thing is, despite all the problems in East Germany, all the Nazis, all the racism (*BIG BIG PROBLEMS*, right, they basically need to defund the East German police, the East German teachers, everyone, it's all fucked), I still think West Germans slag off Easties too much. They slag them off for* EVERYTHING. *As someone who performs at* Lesebühne *(like open-mike reading nights but without the open mike) I often get told afterwards that the others went on about the East too much. "Nobody wants to know about that stuff anymore." But they're often just silly, funny stories about their childhoods. And because the country they grew up in doesn't exist anymore, when they talk about the brands of, I dunno, glue or porridge from their childhoods, they're talking about the East. It reminds me of being a woman: when a woman talks about starting her period, for the first time, maybe, or suddenly on a camping trip, it becomes this hugely feminist story, about her body, about her biology, but in fact she is just talking about her life. (I do wonder if my Lesebühne colleagues from East Germany or East Berlin defend me against the charge of talking about my body too much as much as I do them!)*

Berlin expats still say West Germany, though. And when I say expats, I don't just mean British, American, or Australian newcomers – I mean literally everybody who moves to Berlin without their families: Turkish people, Russian people, Indians, the Thai, the French, the Spanish, the Greeks. For people who arrive in Berlin, there are three regions of Germany: East Germany (full of Nazis), West Germany (boring), and Berlin (good/okay).

Recently a German friend of mine, West German, was over at mine and an expat friend I haven't known very long came over. When my German friend asked my expat friend where she spent

Christmas, she answered "Oh, in West Germany, actually," and my German friend exploded.

"Do you know how hurtful that is?" Katja exploded.

I was a bit embarrassed – like I say, I haven't known this woman, Amya, very long.

"What should I say?" she asked, nonplussed.

"You should specify where you went!" Katja said.

"But why?" I asked. "It can only be Cologne or Hamburg, they're the only two cities in West Germany."

"Do you know how hurtful you are being?" Katja said. "We had to put up with years of being called Wessi, Wessiarsch, Westie, *West German Arsehole. Now even the foreigners laugh at us!"*

"It was Köln," Amya said. "Cologne. Kind of nice there. Not as bad I expected."

I thought Katja was being super precious, to be honest, yeah, people make jokes about West Germans, sometimes – but it's like how British people take the piss out of people who went to Oxford or Cambridge. It's probably a bit annoying when it happens to you, but it's not proper discrimination. East Germans suffer from real discrimination, I think. People laugh at their accents, are snobby about their names – and admit openly to preferring to employ West Germans. I don't think East Germans suffer from racist discrimination. But the Ossi hate is a form of class discrimination which should be less socially acceptable, to be honest.

So, I am not German, which means that my opinion counts for shit, obviously, but I personally wish, wish really hard, that the British way of seeing German reunification was what really happened back then. That two countries, East Germany and West Germany, joined together to form Germany. Taking the best from each country (abortions and Kindergartens in the East, I guess, and freedom of speech and stuff from the West) and created a new country. They could have even named it: Die Vereinigten Staaten von Deutschland, *the United States of Germany.*

Reizwäsche

I am with an East German friend, Jana, in Prenzlauer Berg, when we bump into my ex-husband.

"WHERE'S RYAN?" He screams at me.

"Isn't he with you?" I mutter nonchalantly and watch his head nearly explode.

"He's at Russian Katja's," Jana says, deescalating things. I want my ex-husband to go home so Jana and I can get on with the important business of slagging him off in a feminist manner. Instead, Jana invites him to come and drink cocktails with us, and we all go and get drunker and drunker and drunker (or more and more and more drunk?)

At one point, my German ex-husband says the word "Reizwäsche" at which Jana exclaims: "I always thought you were a Wessi! Jacinta! Your ex-husband is Eastie! He's one of us!"

"Wessis can say *Reizwäsche,*" my ex says sulkily.

"They cannot," Jana says. "They say *sexy Unterwäsche* – sexy underwear."

"I'm not really an Ossi," he says.

"Yeah, I thought you were Swabian!" Jana says.

"We left when I was a kid," he says.

"Oooooooh," Jana says, nodding. "So every now and then you betray yourself!"

There aren't many words left which only Easties say. I mean, it's so many years later, how could there be? East Germany is full of West Germans, and West Germany is full of East Germans. Still. Rule of thumb: Berliners call pancakes *Eierkuchen,* West

Germans call them *Pfannkuchen* and Easties call them *Plinzen.* A *Pfannkuchen* in Berlin is a doughnut, by the way, and not, despite the nice story you learnt in German class, a *Berliner* (sorry). East Berliners and East Germans say *Einraumwohnung,* West Berliners and West Germans say *Einzimmerwohnung,* but remember: they count the living room as a room here, so a two-bedroom flat is a *Dreizimmerwohnung*! Westies say *Supermarkt* and Easties say *Kaufhalle.* West Germans say "Ich habe *Bärenhunger*" and Easties say "Ich habe *Knast*". Some people say that saying "Leo seine Sachen" for Leo's things is an East German thing, but I am not so sure. I have definitely met a lot of East Germans who say it, but quite a few West Germans, too. It seems to be dying out as a mistake, too, or maybe my German-speaking friends are just posher than they were a few years ago!

* * *

Wiebke: *One of the weirdest things about living in a different country to the one you grew up in, is that you automatically become a bit less snobby (well most people do, the most dire snobs stay as snobby as ever, but just in two different languages/cultures). Because lots of things you have always thought were posh are considered working class, and lots of things you think are a bit common are considered perfectly fine.*

And it takes you ages to work out which names are "bad" or not. You can't even tell which names are young or not.

I used to think the German Karen was called Wiebke, but that doesn't mean I thought Wiebkes were like Karens. I thought they were softer, more annoying, better educated – but super white and always buying organic. I've changed my mind, though, since writing this column. I now think the German Karen is actually called Jana – and Wiebke is more like a Becky.

The last kid who came to my house before Corona times was a quiet, serious boy with a glamorous, almost flamboyant mum, Nadine. Nadine's about ten years younger than me and looks like the richest girl in my year at school so I sometimes get a bit mixed up in my head and act like I've known her for years and years – when I actually met her last summer.

So, in February, before Corona times started coronaing, Nadine phones me up – being ten years younger than me, of course, she sent me a WhatsApp message beforehand, asking if she could – and then announced, flamboyantly, glamorously, that she wanted to go to the cinema. Actually, I think she said "movies".

"I really want to go to the movies!" she said.

I wasn't sure if she was inviting me to the cinema with her or not. She's a very flamboyant, glamorous person, you know, the kind of person who would hot-foot it to the cinema after Kita – with a couple of toddlers in tow.

"Baby Leo's not been to the cinema yet," I said cautiously. I am not a hugely cautious person, I don't think, but I am not super-glam either. "Just the Lego 4D cinema at the *Legoland Discovery Center*. He got a bit scared during the police chase."

"Well," she said, "I was thinking I could drop Laurence off at yours around seven, come pick him after the movies, or maybe I could even sleep at yours, shall I bring you some popcorn?"

"Don't bring me any popcorn," I said sadly. "I'm meant to be be ketoing."

"I could bring you some plain popcorn? Salty popcorn?'" she said.

"Plain popcorn isn't keto either," I said, even more sadly.

"Are you sure?" she asked. "It's just corn, isn't it? It's just a vegetable?"

"Yeah, I'm sure," I said, sadder than ever. People in their early 30s have some very optimistic ideas about keto.

So Laurence, her grave, funny boy, stayed over. He's one of those kids where everything they say is a sudden, serious announcement.

"I can't sleep!" he announced suddenly, in his serious little voice. "I'm worried about Karius and Baktus."

He didn't have his toothbrush with him, and I couldn't find a spare one, and German kids worry a lot about Karius and Baktus.

"I don't think Karius and Baktus come every night," I said.

He sat up in the mini-bed I'd fashioned for him out of cushions on the floor.

"I think they do, actually."

Baby Leo toddled, waddled, into the room. Compared to Laurence, he was 100 per cent toddler – his fat bum, swaddled in his nappy, gave him a Donald Duck vibe, his fat, sturdy turkey legs made him look like a little Buddha. He pointed at Laurence's impromptu cushion bed.

"Ich auch!" He shouted happily and the boys burst out laughing. By the time they fell asleep, it was 11.50 pm, and the next day there was going to be a big costume party at Kita – an incredibly early *Fasching*. I remember looking at the clock and thinking, imagine if I was German – imagine if I was called Wiebke – I'd never agree to this.

Nadine's German, but she's not GERMAN-German. She's not a Wiebke. Wiebke is kind of like a German Karen, although the analogy isn't great – Wiebkes are softer than Karens, give their kids homeopathic medicines for teething, for example, but take them to the real doctor's when they break a leg. Wiebkes boycott Disney, never go to *Legoland* because of the sensory overload, eat tofu paté for dinner, and, most importantly of all: ALWAYS GET THEIR KIDS INTO BED BY 7 pm.

Imagine dropping your kid off at 7 pm at a Wiebke's – just so you could go to the pictures. They'd literally die – their brains would explode, their hearts implode, their internal organs would fail, their lungs would collapse like they were the World Trade Center lined with explosives.

I'm not friends with many Wiebkes. I don't see how you can be – when would you meet up? Their kids have their midday sleep at 12:30, sleep until 1:30 or maybe 2:00 p.m. Any activity you'd play has to be over by 5.30 pm AT THE ABSOLUTE LATEST so the kids can have their tofu paté dinner at 6 pm – and be tucked up in bed by 7.

You think I am slagging the Wiebkes off, but I'm not, not really. Well, okay, I am, but I don't mean it as harshly as it might sound. I am a mum, I know kids, I know how anstrengend they are. I know men, I know how lazy they can be, I know motherhood, I know how exhausting it can get. I believe Wiebke when she says her kids have to be asleep by seven. I respect 7 pm bedtimes – Baby Leo has been in bed by seven so many times – I know how gorgeous it feels, to have hours and hours of literal freedom stretched out in front of you, even if you do end up filling it all up with cleaning the kitchen and watching Netflix.

This is what I don't understand. I can't totally understand how Wiebkes don't find time spent with other people SO MUCH FUN that every now and again they buy a bottle of cheap white wine and go to a friend's house, shut the Kinderzimmer door and let the kids stay up till midnight. And I also can't understand why Wiebkes have suddenly discovered how important socialising is. Like I would've expected the glamorously flamboyant types like Nadine to think life without socialising not worth living. But it's the Wiebkes who are complaining the loudest! People who only organise social activities with other people for a fixed window of 2.5 hours in the middle of the afternoon now think their kids are so traumatised by lack of social contact? How do they even notice the difference?

All the Wiebkes I know are writing 3000-word status updates about how awful the lack of social contact is for their kids.

I don't know. I kind of feel like playdates, those parcels of time, those artificial slices of social contact, are actually slightly more depressing and lonely than three months of hermiting yourself away with your kid, but I guess it's just me.

Baby Leo and I walked past a super-full playground the other day.

"Schlayschound," he said, which is how he, horrifically, pronounces the word "playground", "is. Nicht. Mehr. Kaputt-Schlayschound is better."

"Yeah," I said. "They opened up the playgrounds again."

"Playground. Is. Nice." He said. And then he looked at me questioningly: "Hein?" This is, reasonably enough, how he pronounces the word *rein*.

"Better not," I said. "Look how full it is. Let's go play on the grass with the football."

"Okaaaaaaaay," he said cheerfully, and I wondered if I had swapped places with Wiebke. Wiebke, with her DM sunblock and her Regenhose, is now the fearless one, who thinks social interactions are more important than anything else.

Chapter Twenty-Four: X is for ...

XL: *So, I don't know why this is, but when you go to coffee shops, they literally never talk about the sizes of their cups in German. It might be in Italian – venti, etc – or it might be in English. And what they literally never ever do is shorten* klein, mittel, groß *to K, M, G. I don't know why? It's always S, M, L, XL. Maybe they think KMG are just kind of boring letters, which I guess is kind of true.*

They also call coffees that you take away Kaffee ToGo *but watch out, you have to pronounce it like an East German grandma talking about the country Torgorrr – if you say it normally, they'll switch to English. I've said* zu gehen *on a number of occasions and nobody ever corrected me.*

Body Positivity

In my woke German/Berlin bubble, lots of middle-class white people talk all this theoretical, idealistic stuff about body positivity. But everyone weighs exactly 48 kilos and has perfect hair and the flattest stomachs you have ever seen. Especially German women who have just given birth, by the way. The flatter a German woman's stomach, the more recently she just gave birth. I don't know what's wrong with these people sometimes!

So my woke leftist German friends talk the body positivity talk but they walk, and I mean this in the nicest, most respectful, feminist way possible, a skinny bitch walk.

And when I go home to Britain, I just think: God you guys have so much to teach us. In the UK, working class women, of whatever size, and I mean WHATEVER size, just put on mini skirts when they want to feel sexy. And then, at 11 o'clock at night, they spill out of the pubs onto the pavement outside, and they spill out of their spaghetti strapped dresses and yeah, yeah, yeah. They eat too much, maybe, and drink too much, almost definitely, and they also go to the tanning salons too often and they haven't completely resolved all this trauma from their past – but there's also such joy there, such love, as they fall out of their clothes and fall down onto the floor. I watch them now, like a German tourist, my eyes soaking them up, my body filled with envy, disapproval, and also desire. They're so free, and my body positivity is so theoretical. We have so much to learn from them.

Chapter Twenty-Five: Y is for …

You: Du, Ihr *or* Sie.

I'm guessing you guys remember, somewhat traumatisedly, that there are approximately one squillion words for "the" in the German language. Unfortunately, there's quite a few for "you" too.

Du *is the informal one – the one you use for friends or kids. It's* du *in the nominative,* dich *in the accusative,* dir *in the dative.* Du liebst mich, ich liebe dich, ich gebe dir ein Geschenk. *Watch out, though: this is only singular. You have to be one-on-one to use this* du.

Ihr *is what you say to a classroom full of kids or a Bachelor-Party of drunk lads at Alexanderplatz:* Ihr seid Arschlöcher, ich hasse euch, ich gebe euch eine Klatsche, wenn ihr mir zu nah kommt. *It's the plural informal.*

Sie *is what you say to your boss or elderly people. Confusingly, it can be singular OR plural. It's* Sie *in the nominative, accusative, and* Ihnen *in the dative.* Kommen Sie mit! Ich sehe Sie da. Ich erkläre es Ihnen. *This is the same word as "they – but capitalised! –" When I first lived in Germany, I had a job in an ice cream café, and every time the other ladies asked the customers "Was bekommen Sie denn?" or "Wie kann ich Ihnen helfen?" I'd think they were speaking to me and say, shruggingly, "I dunno, just ask them." A weird thing about* Sie *is that people who get into a verbal fight with each other can say* "Arschloch" *to each other without switching to*

Sie. *So, even though it is rude to say* du *to a stranger, you'll even hear people saying "Sie sind ein Arschloch!" every now and again.*

Another weird thing is, when I came to Germany, I thought there were too many words for "you" but after twenty-one years, I think there aren't enough! I think we need a plural for Sie – Sies *would do nicely, I think – and we also need a hybrid for* Sie/euch *for parents' evenings at schools and theatre shows where there are lots of students, but also lots of older people, in the audience – I'd suggest* seuch.

When you say du *to someone, you're* duzing *them, and when you say* Sie *to someone, you're* siezing *them. Weirdly you never* ihrzen *or* euchzen *people, though. I guess you're just duzing them in plural? In Berlin, we generally duzen a bit more freely than in other places in Germany. We duzen our neighbours a lot, for example, or parents will usually duzen the teachers at the Kita.*

People often wrongly think that in English there's no word for Sie – that we're all duzing each other – but in fact, this isn't true. It's the du *form which is missing – thou was the old* du *form, something which is quite obvious when you think about it – compare* thou hast *with* du hast *and it makes complete sense that* thou *and* du *are connected. However, the thing is, a language where there is no distinction between formal and informal you automatically seems a bit more informal. Look at the way nurses and doctors will call their patients by their first names in the UK and the US and I think you can see that if we could duzen, we would!*

I don't really miss Sie *when speaking English to English speakers – but sometimes if there is an older German I speak English to, I feel a bit ashamed to say the word "you" to them. It rhymes with* du *and it just seems so bald and naked. Sometimes, when teaching TEFL to an older German, I'll try and avoid the word "you" altogether and create weird sentences like "And the homework for this week ... is it finished?" "Have you done your homework?" sounds a bit like "Hast du deine Hausaufgaben gemacht?" and just feels a bit ... disrespectful.*

The word I miss, even when speaking English to English speakers, is ihr/euch. *It's just lovely to have a grammatically correct way of addressing more than one person at the same time! It's so obviously missing in the English language. The Scottish and Londoners have just corrected the mistake by brazenly adding se onto you and Americans have their brilliant y'all – they can even turn it into a possessive pronoun "Have y'all done y'all's homework?"*

Don't get me wrong, none of this is grammatically correct – but it is necessary. Standard English is just incomplete, basically. When my oldest son was little and had a friend over for dinner, I was forced to speak incorrectly, because whenever I said "You can have ice-cream later!" he would start crying and say "WHAT ABOUT ME?!?"

"Youse can both have ice-cream," I'd clarify. What choice did I have?

Sprechen Sie Englisch?

Slightly depressingly, when my little brother visited me in Neukölln shortly before the pandemic started, the thing which marked him out as a tourist was that he asked, when entering the Spätis: "Sprechen Sie Englisch?" before communicating with the *Spätibetreiber.*

"You don't need to ask them if they can speak English," my son told him. "They all do. And if you do ask them, you should say *Sprichst du Englisch?* not *Sprechen Sie Englisch?*"

"No, Ryan," I said sternly. "You should say *Sie* to a shopworker."

"Yeah but not a Späti guy," my son said. We started arguing about whether saying *Sie* or *Du* to Späti people was rude or not.

"Bakeries are Sie, pharmacies are Sie, Media Markt is Sie," my son said. "Spätis are du places. Especially Spätis in Neukölln."

"I dunno," I said.

"Even if you do say Sie to them, they say du back to you," Ryan said.

"Well, they can say du to you!" I said with great gusto. "You're just a kid!"

It says something about the level of modern language teaching in Great Britain that my brother actually learnt German up to the age of fifteen without ever having learnt the difference between Sie and du – or maybe he had just forgotten the distinction in the ten years since leaving school.

"There's a different word for you if you're talking to a kid?" my brother asked.

I tried to explain the whole difference to him, and it was kind of complicated. We got on the bus and sat at the top and tried to go over the differences.

"Kids are always du, and animals too," my son explained. "But some teachers are du, the nicest ones. Mean teachers are Sie."

"It's just a thing we do in German," I said. "It's more polite. It's more respectful."

My brother was aghast.

"Are you saying kids don't need respect?"

"Well, no, but ..."

"Are you saying kids are like animals?"

"Look, it's just like ... it's more respectful to call a grown-up Sie. But it's not disrespectful to call a kid du. It's like, I'd never call a baby Sir or Madam. Right?"

My brother remained horrified.

"And there are teachers you say Sie to and they say du to you back?" He looked at my son and then at me. "Sis, this isn't okay! You have to do something about it. Write a column about it, tweet about it – you have loads of followers. Get people angry! Kids deserve respect, and they don't deserve to be spoken to like animals."

"No, it's ... it's fine. I don't mind people saying du to Ryan. It's okay."

"You think it's okay?"

"It's not a political issue. Like, it can be. The controllers on the U-Bahn say du to homeless people and refugees too much. I've tweeted the BVG about it before. But it's fine for the kids, you couldn't say Sie to a kid. It would be too ... awkward."

"You think refugees deserve respect but kids don't! Sis, I'm so surprised at you."

"It's not really about respect. It's like distance. It puts distance between you, like when a nurse says, how are we feeling. Because it really means they, you know? I dunno. It's hard to understand if you can't speak German."

"You should go into school and say I want to be spoken to with respect," my brother told my son.

We sat in silence. I didn't really know how to get him to understand the difference between du and Sie, and that while it's not okay to say du to a refugee, nobody would ever siezen a baby. Even ironically siezing a baby would feel weird. *Ich muss Ihnen jetzt die Windel wechseln.* May I change your nappy, dear Sir?

"They say du to God," I said, after a few minutes' silence. "It's not just kids and animals and refugees and the homeless and your friends. It's God, too. When Germans pray, they say du to God."

"Well, if I was God I would be really fucking pissed off about that," my brother answered. "I bet when Germans die and go to Heaven, the first thing God tells them to do is to call him Sie."

Chapter Twenty-Six: Z is for …

Zecke: Zecke *means tick, but also a left-wing person, possibly a squatter/hippy/punk type person.*

Where the Ticks Come From

I once told a German colleague I lived in Friedrichshain and she said: "Da kommen die Zecken her!" "That's where the ticks came from!" and I said "That's funny. We don't have much woodland, to be honest."

* * *

Zug: Zug *means train, but also draught. Weirdly, overdrawn is* überzogen *– but overdraft is not* Überzug *but* Dispo.

The Mystery of the Poisonous Sook

When my oldest boy was born, we lived in a women's refuge, and he had a lot of eye infections, chest infections and was just generally a sickly, poorly little thing. (His little brother, who I didn't breastfeed, not even for a second, got ill once during his first year on this earth, like a hearty, stout peasant, whereas Ryan was constantly, constantly sick. This is not me saying breastfeeding is worthless. Maybe if Ryan hadn't been breastfed, he would have got ill even more often, and maybe, had Leo been breastfed, he would have made it through the first year without even being ill once. But it does make me wonder if the wonders of breastfeeding get a tiny bit exaggerated sometimes?)

The other mums in the refuge told me where these illnesses came from. It came from a terrible chemical in the walls, "sook." I thought it was a chemical in the walls, but sometimes I thought it was a chemical that it was in clouds all over Berlin, sweeping across the city, like smog. Even though our refuge was in West Berlin, I thought it was an East thing. Chemicals from factories they'd had there once. Which they'd never managed to completely eradicate.

It wasn't just the other mums in the refuge though. Even grannies on the U-Bahn, or in the street, came up to me and warned me about the sook. His eyes were all caked up with goo or gunk and a granny would nod wisely and say savagely "It's the sook. It gets in through the windows."

It seemed to be everywhere.

One day I went to the Jugendamt, to the Unterhaltsvorschusskasse, and the baby coughed.

"I hope he isn't getting ill again," I said to the case worker.

"It's the sook," she said wisely.

"Yes, because our building our women's refuge is full of sook," I told her. "You'd think they'd do something about it."

"There's not much they can do about it," she said. "All old buildings have it. It's even here, in the Jugendamt."

"EVEN HERE!" I wailed. The one place in Berlin I thought would be free of sook was, surely, the Jugendamt? I imagined this invisible asbestos-like chemical circling the old building, creeping in through the windows and descending down upon my baby and entering his eyes.

It was pretty scary for a young mum, as you can imagine. And the other thing you have to remember is that we didn't have Google on our phones. There was all this stuff we didn't know, and couldn't google. The English translation for sook fell into this category.

When Ryan was eleven months old, we went home to the UK. I stayed in my parents' house (sook-free at last!) for a month. While there, I gave up breastfeeding – everyone in Britain praised me so much for having breastfed for so long that I felt like a bit of a mug, to be honest – and listened to my mum's advice about sleep-training and felt very confused. "He needs to know who's boss!" she explained. "But how does him lying there, screaming in agony, and me lying there, suffering in silence in agony, make him think I am the boss?" I asked, genuinely confused. But we did clear one thing up: The Mystery of the Poisonous Sook.

"It's a chemical that's still in all German buildings, it is outside in the streets, it's everywhere," I said. "It's worse in wintertime, but it's bad in summer too. It gives babies chest infections, eye infections, but it can also give grannies shoulder ache."

"It sounds awful."

"And we don't have it in London?" my sister asked

"Some people told me we must do, it's all over the world, but I never heard of it."

"If it's making people so sick, you'd think the government would do something about it."

"They literally can't do anything about it. The whole city is poisoned. It's made Ryan so ill, it caused all the illnesses he had. Well, the doctor said he might have got them anyway, but the sook didn't help."

"Let's look it up in the dictionary. See what it says."

But when we looked up the word, sook, we couldn't find anything. I was really surprised.

"I'll send my friend a text message and check exactly how it's spelt."

So I texted my women's refuge bestie (we weren't saying bestie yet, mind) Russian Katja and asked her: "Katja, wie buchstabiert man *Sook*, weißt du, dieses Ding, das die Kinder krank macht?" She wrote back: "Zug." I wrote back: "Dasselbe Wort wie Bahn? Zug?" And then we looked it up in the big, big German-English dictionary.

"Procession, parade, line, stream, march, passage, movement, drift, journey, passage, flock, school, shoal, catch, haul, team, platoon, convoy, mountain range, row, draft, draught, puff, drag, pull, breath, draft (drink), draught (drink), mouthful, swig."

"I can't see any chemicals here, Cinty," my mum said, almost crossly, but mostly kindly. I stared at the dictionary page in confusion.

"I'll text a German," I said. "Katja isn't a native speaker. Her real name isn't even Katja."

My mum coughed politely.

"Some old people," she said, "sometimes think that draughty houses give them shoulder pains."

I stared at her and slowly realised what had happened.

It's a sign of how much my family loved me and Ryan that they never took the piss out of me for having thought, for a whole year, that Berlin was so polluted with ancient DDR factory chemicals that just going out the house could make you ill. They were mostly relieved that the walls of the old houses in Berlin weren't infected with a type of asbestos nobody outside of Germany had ever heard of before, as, it must be said, was I.

Epilogue: Why You Should Learn German and Some Tips on How to

My mum used to say you knew you were getting old, when you noticed how young policemen looked. I think for me, it's more true: I knew I was getting old when, every time I met a Berlin mum under 30, I assumed she was a teenie mama.

So, I met a British single mum at a playground in Lichtenberg the other day.

"How old are you?" I asked her. "You look about twelve."

"I'm 26," she said.

I gasped in horror. "You poor thing. A single mum – and so young – and your baby is so young – and your family are all in Britain and you don't even have a man to rely on!" I looked at her with so much pity. "What are you going to do? How are you going to cope? Have you told the Jugendamt you need help? You're so young, you're so vulnerable, how is anyone ever meant to cope in a position like this?"

Suddenly, I remembered that I had been in exactly the same position she was in now, all those years ago, back when Tempelhof was still a running airport and all the Nettos were called Plus. It hadn't seemed that bad at all. It had been kind of fun. I can't remember much, but I don't think things were that unbearably horrific to tell you the truth.

We sat at the side of the empty playground, shivering, and made small talk.

"Don't you think the Germans wrap their kids up too warm?" she asked me. "Like, just because it's winter, doesn't mean it's *Games of Thrones*-type weather? They always insist on the kids wearing hats and scarves and gloves and a thousand pullovers. And they keep the heating on too high in the Kitas? This is why their kids are always getting sick! Libby hasn't been sick once this year. I come from a family who live in a really draughty old house, you know."

Something about the way she said the words "family" and "really draughty old house" made me decide she was secretly an aristocrat and had grown up in a stately home.

"That's something I could blog about," I said.

Her face turned to stone.

"Do you blog for Exberliner?" she asked.

"Yes," I said. I could tell she was, like, physically shaken, visibly paled, all that sort of stuff.

"Your rant made me cry," she whispered bleakly, and honestly, I don't think I have ever felt more guilty about anything in my whole life ever.

"Which one?" I whispered back even more bleakly.

"The German one," she said. I took in a deep breath. "The German one?" I asked incredulously. "Are you sure you read it properly?"

"I KNOW I should learn German," she said, breathlessly. "I know I should. And I know I would, if I tried to. Well, I think I would. But I just don't have any money – I have no money – I am a single mother on benefits!" she exclaimed, looking at me angrily. Secretly I added the words with an aristocratic family who all live in a mansion in my head. "If I have any money left over from raising my child," she paused dramatically, "I spend it on things that are, you know, good for my mental health. I don't think paying for a babysitter and a Volkshochschule course and then spending, like, Thursday night struggling with *der die* and *das* would be very good for my mental health!"

"No," I agreed. "It sounds like that would be terrible for your mental health."

"And I don't have the money at the moment."

"You shouldn't have cried," I said feebly. She was really pretty, and blonde, and delicate – fragile and delicate and porcelain and weak. "It wasn't having a go at people like you. It was having a go at arrogant men. Not people like you. You're not arrogant about it. You see not being able to speak German as a failure." Which it KIND OF is, I added secretly in my head, but not out loud. I didn't want her to start crying right there in the playground.

"It made me cry for half an hour," she said.

"Blimey," I said and sat there and thought about what I had done and how I could make amends.

So: this is the thing. I am so fucking *priviligiert* on the German-speaking scale, the only people more privileged than me are people who are naturally good at languages and grammar and accents and stuff (PUKE) and those secret bilinguals you meet at parties sometimes and they pretend to come from Dorset but it turns out their dad comes from Dorset, they spent a year there when they were four, but they actually grew up in Hamburg. We've all met them. I know I am privileged, I have German GCSE, German A-Level, a German Bachelor's, I have lived here for half my actual life and my entire adult life, I have two German-speaking (more or less) kids and I am, basically, practically German now. I don't want to make any less privileged people cry, this is the opposite of everything I want to achieve in life and through writing.

BUT (it's a Nicki Minaj size butt) I do think you should learn German. I'm not going to bullshit you. There is no need to learn German just so you can speak to waiters or shop assistants in German. We all know you get better service if they think you're a posh expat rather than a poor immigrant. Also, you also don't really need to learn German to speak to doctors – they can all speak English now. You also won't make more friends in Germany if you speak German – everyone 40 and under is better at English than you will ever, ever be in German. You also are never going to read "Effi Briest" or "Faust" or whatever, and even if you do decide to go to the theatre you can just go on the nights when they have surtitles on.

You should learn German because:

1. IT'S FUN. It's hard and it's annoying and after seventy-four years here you'll find out that shoelaces are *Schnürsenkel* and not *Schuhschnekel* (WHY?) but there are lots of fun things you can say in German. Words that are literally fun to say in your mouth. The most fun thing about German is the making up of long words. Germans do this themselves – *Backpfeifengesicht*, for example, someone just made that up one day, and now it's in the dictionary– but you can make up your own ones, too. *Unterhaltsvorschussproblematiküberwältigungsfeiergrund*, for example: which is the word for when you finally get a back payment on child support advance payments and invite everyone you know to the pub to get wasted.

2. Talking to grannies. The problem with grannies in Germany is they're fucking MEAN but if you ever want to talk to any of these mean German grannies, you better learn some German.

3. Talking to taxi drivers. There are some taxi drivers who speak English but the best *Taxigespräche* are always, always, ALWAYS in German.

4. Talking to Easties: When I say Easties, I mean people who were twenty and over when the wall fell. You'll need to learn German if you want to get the really good gossip about how

the Stasi confiscated their walkmen and what they spent their *Begrüßungsgeld* on and stuff.

5. German films, by which I mean, of course, *Lola Rennt* and *Goodbye Lenin*.

6. If you have kids, you'll need to learn German for when their friends come over. You need to warn them about Karies and Baktus, and you'll want to be able to understand what they're saying when they're fighting.

7. Going to Amts: I think of Amts in Berlin as like the Asterix village of the German language now.

8. When people in the street insult you, it's very satisfying to be able to insult them back in German, it's also slightly more satisfying to start crying and explain how sad they've made you and watch them curl up with disgust and fear.

9. Emergencies: let's be honest, you don't need German at the doctor, but you do/might need it if you call the cops.

10. In-laws: if you manage to snag yourself a German partner, you'll probably need to speak a bit of German here. They'll like you more if you at least try.

Okay so that's the why, here's the how:

1. First up, there's this 100 per cent totally free course you can do online with *Deutsche Welle*: there are videos, audios, podcasts – and classes ranging from A1 to C!

2. Second up – sign up for the e-mail course at *Learn German with Oliver*! Oliver will send you daily exercises, written texts and apparently addictive online games. Why not spend that time you waste on *Angry Birds* on the U-Bahn improving your German skills

2. Watch dubbed movies. I am not a sociopath – I know you're not about to go and watch *Last Christmas* in German, or put the *Marriage Story* or *Working Moms* on in German. I mean, the only way I would ever ever EVER do this is if I

fell in love with some non-German person (not being racist, I am imagining a Mongolian here) who for some reason had an eye infection and couldn't read subtitles and he was really, really, REALLY good-looking and there were no German movies on for us to go and see. MAYBE. I am not suggesting you do anything WEIRD and UNNATURAL and BARBARIC and HORRIFICALLY DISGUSTING here. But – if you have kids, you can go and watch shitty cartoons in German, can't you. And by shitty cartoons I do not mean *Frozen 2*, obviously, I mean *Cars* and stuff. AND: you can watch all your old favourite movies – the kind of films you know off by heart – *Dirty Dancing, Pretty Woman, Home Alone, Blink* in German. Just for fun, I am not sure if fun is the right word. Watch *Dirty Dancing* in German with English subtitles. Then watch it in German, with German subtitles. Then watch it in German WITH NO SUBTITLES. Okay this might sound like a bit of a basic hobbylose activity but let me tell you, when you are done, you will be able to say "ich habe eine Wassermelone getragen" like a pro.

4. Watch German stuff. I know, I know. It's hard and it's depressing. The trouble is, any German stuff which is actually artistically worth watching is linguistically pretty highbrow and often a lot of the characters have cancer and/or get betrayed to the Stasi by their families. I personally think if you want to learn German, you should watch one tacky reality TV show/ soap a day. I am sorry for being such a Basic Betty here. They are AWFUL. In a way I find those tacky shows on German TV worse than the British or the US-American ones, because the English-speaking ones are all about how can we bitchily yet subtly suggest that you're not quite good enough, whereas the German ones everyone just spends the whole time going: "Das geht gar nicht, soll das ein Geburtstagskuchen sein?" But the language is simple enough for you to follow, and the central conceit of the shows is always so clear and simple to grab hold

of that you can use logic to make up for what you're lacking in linguistic comprehension. If you watch German TV online, like on the official ARD website, you can put subtitles on, by the way. And of course Netflixers have subtitle options too. A show I really liked – I didn't love it, but I really enjoyed it – was *Dogs of Berlin*. It was fast in a way German shows often aren't, and a bit silly at times, and relatively unjudgey.

5. Give yourself a new word to try out each day – or even seven. Try and shoe-horn random German words into a sentence and say it to a stranger in the street or a neighbour or a German mum at the Kita. Your word for today is *Backpfeifengesicht* – the kind of face you just have to slap.

6. Integration courses. This tip is only free if you are on Hartz IV, otherwise, they give you half your money back when you pass the integration test. Contact BAMS to find out the integration course nearest to you. Warning (I know this from a friend of mine who did one) they will tell you that the German flag is black, red and gold. IT IS NOT GOLD, IT IS A HORRIBLE YELLOW.

7. Don't worry about grammar, fuck that shit. Honestly, either you're good at grammar, in which case you don't need to worry about it, or you're like the rest of us, and it's totally hard, and you'll never get good at it. Fuck it, man. I once interviewed a little old Turkish lady who had lived here since she was twenty and been evicted from her flat and I don't think she got one of her *ders, dies* or *dasses* right the whole interview but you know what IT DIDN'T MATTER HER GERMAN WAS BRILLIANT SHE WAS BILINGUAL. Don't worry about grammar. It's meaningless. Germans are never going to use the present, perfect or continuous properly and we are never going to remember when you say *das Teil* and when it's *der Teil* and it literally could not matter less all you need to do is get those words out your mouth, baby.

8. Put on the radio. There's not just telly, you know. Put the radio on and half-listen. Do the washing up. One day, when you're bored, you'll listen more. And then one day, when you didn't even notice you were that bored, you'll suddenly notice you listened to an entire documentary about Ernst Thälmann and okay maybe you didn't understand every word but you kind of understood every sentence. And that, my friends, is a beautiful feeling.

9. Duolingo. I don't need to explain too much here. That owl's a bit of a smug cunt, though.

10. (This is the hardest bit.) Read in German. Don't read anything too hard, or the words will just close up like you're Sylvia Plath and the German language is enclosed in a *Dornröschen* thorn bush of impenetrable black letters. Don't read anything written before the late 20th century, except Kafka. Kafka's good. Read (don't kill me here) read the *B.Z.* and the *Berliner Kurier.* Unlike the UK equivalents, the *Sun* and the *Mirror,* these are written so that people with limited language skills can read them, there's hardly ever any crazy puns or weird rhymes and alliteration. Please take everything they say about *Laternenfest* with a pinch of salt, they have to sell papers somehow. If you are too left-wing/cool for skool and you would rather die than read a proper tabloid, you can read *taz* in simple language, go to the bottom of their website and click *in einfacher Sprache.* If you're a bit of a gossip girl, read *InTouch* magazine. Try to read *Spiegel,* but not too much. You don't want to get a headache. I wouldn't want to make you cry.

Come on you guys – you can do it. Or, as we say in German: Ihr schafft das schon!

Glossary

Here are some of the German words used in this book which you might not have learnt yet: I've translated them for you, so there's no need to google!

Alexa: best shopping centre in Berlin, it's really good

Alice Schwarzer: one of Germany's leading feminists, getting a bit racist and transphobic in her old age though

angesprochen: addressed/spoken to

Apfelschorle: wonderfully delicious apple juice mixed with sparkling water. See also *Weißweinschorle*. Apparently Germans living in Britain miss bread loads, but I think I'd miss all the Schorles*.

Bescheid wissen: to know. Like to really know. TO KNOW. If you know, you know. And if you KNOW, you weißt Bescheid

BSR: the company that picks up your rubbish in Berlin. They even do a sexy calendar at Christmas

Dönerladen: Kebab shop, yum

Eckkneipe: Old Man's Pub, but on a corner

Erlebnis: experience

* The correct plural is "Schorlen". — Last note of the German editor

Faschingskostüm: Fasching is German Pancake Day, only they dress up for it, yay. *Faschingskostüm* is the costume kids put on for Fasching. German kids are so spoilt, they basically get to dress up for Fasching AND Halloween. Also spare a thought for Anglo expat housewives living in Germany/Berlin who have to spend the morning painting faces and the evening flipping pancakes, you guys, the double mental load is REAL

Frauenhaus: a women's shelter

fortschrittliche Kreise: posh, intellectual circles

gefühlsbetont: emotive

Gemeinsam: together

Glatt (glatter): smoooooooooooooth

Kampfhund: scary dogs that Nazis like

Kindergeburtstag: child's birthday (party)

Kontrolleur: Like ticket inspectors, but total thugs, because it's super easy to get on the train without a ticket, so the whole point is they're meant to catch you

Laternenfest: really boring German version of Halloween with no candy, no costumes, and there's lanterns, but the lanterns are just shit and boring and not in pumpkins. Every year Bild gets really upset about how it's dying out and they blame the Muslims but really they should just blame German kids wanting candy and costumes and actual FUN for once in their miserable German lives

Meldepflicht: you can't translate this word! The legal requirement to register your address with the local authorities (so weird)

Mischling: for dogs, it means mongrel, but it is sometimes used, sadly, as a disparaging term for mixed-race people (and sometimes ironically by mixed-raced people themselves, because, also sadly, there aren't really any good words to describe mixed-race people)

Muschi: pssy, but not quite as porny a word. Like you can say it to your kid. If you have to

Pipifax: something really unimportant and trivial

Religionsunterricht: RE class

Schulpflicht: another word that is impossible to translate. The legal requirement to send your kids to school. The weird thing about German *Schulpflicht* is that, in non-pandemic times, homeschooling is illegal. So you literally HAVE to send your kid to school. They don't even let people go on holiday!

Seepferdchen: Swimming certificate kids get. Literally "little sea horse"

Senat: Berlin city government

Spaßbad: really brilliant swimming pool, with a wave machine

Stasi-Vergangenheit: Stasi past (*Stasi* = *Staatssicherheit.* DDR's secret service)

Stasi-Tante: Stasi lady

steil: steep

Stau: traffic jam

Tankstelle: petrol station

Tierheim: animal shelter

Tropical Islands: brilliant but very expensive swimming pool/ fake beach resort

übertrieben: OTT

Unkraut: weeds

Volkshochschule: people's high school, but not in a North Korea kinda way. It's like an adult education centre, basically

Winnetou: Karl May's Indian chief

Danke schön & THANKS THANKS THANKS go to:

Volker, the strictest German editor in the world, Ruby Russell & Phil Butland, for all their help and advice, encouragement and support, Nadja Vancauwenberghe, the one who started everything in the WTF Berlin universe and, last but not least, Elliot Hermann who taught me the truth about Berlin house numbers. And I also want to thank Jake Schneider and Julia Naji, for always inspiring me to think about language, and of course L and R, my darling boys, who can never understand why my German is so bad, but love me anyway – I LOVE YOU BOYS!